THE
ACID
ALKALINE
FOOD GUIDE

A QUICK REFERENCE TO FOODS
& THEIR EFFECT ON pH LEVELS

DR. SUSAN E. BROWN
LARRY TRIVIERI, Jr.

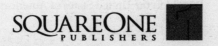

SQUAREONE
PUBLISHERS

The information and advice contained in this book are based upon the research and the personal and professional experiences of the authors. They are not intended as a substitute for consulting with a health care professional. The publisher and authors are not responsible for any adverse effects or consequences resulting from the use of any of the suggestions, preparations, or procedures discussed in this book. All matters pertaining to your physical health should be supervised by a health care professional. It is a sign of wisdom, not cowardice, to seek a second or third opinion.

COVER DESIGNER: Jeannie Tudor
IN-HOUSE EDITOR: Joanne Abrams
TYPESETTER: Gary A. Rosenberg

Square One Publishers
115 Herricks Road • Garden City Park, NY 11040
516-535-2010 • 877-900-BOOK
www.SquareOnePublishers.com

ISBN 0-7570-0280-3
ISBN 978-0-7570-0280-0

CONTENTS

ACKNOWLEDGMENTS

In particular, I acknowledge Dr. Russell Jaffe, Director of ELISA/ACT Biotechnologies, for his scientific and clinically proven work calculating the acid and alkaline impact of foods. His tireless efforts to teach others the "Alkaline Way" diet and lifestyle have contributed to health restoration for thousands of individuals. It was my great privilege to work with Dr. Jaffe, teaching his very successful ELISA/ACT LRA Program for health recovery, and to learn from him firsthand the tremendous clinical value of restoring pH balance. Over two decades ago, Dr. Jaffe led the way in researching and developing a comprehensive, yet simple, classification of foods according to their impact on metabolic acid-alkaline balance.

My work has also been influenced and uplifted by the new wave of scientists studying chronic low-grade metabolic acidosis and its impact on a variety of health concerns, ranging from osteoporosis and kidney stones to muscle loss. These forward-looking researchers to whom I am indebted include Dr. Lynda Frassetto and her colleagues at the University of California, San Francisco, and Dr. Susan New at the University of Surrey, UK. From the European arena, I acknowledge in particular the ground-breaking work of German researchers Drs. Thomas Remer and Friedrich Manz in proposing a formula for calculating the acid-base impact of foods. Some of their research findings are used in this book. Additionally, I congratulate Dr. Jurgen Vormann of the Institute for Prevention and Nutrition in Ismaning, Germany, for his efforts in gathering together the worldwide scientific community engaged in the study of chronic low-grade metabolic acidosis.

I also acknowledge and appreciate the teachings of macrobiotic leader Herman Aihara and his students. In particular, I would like to thank David Briscoe for sharing his insights and encouragement. I thank those closest to home: my clients; my assistant, Janet; my son, Michael; and my partner, Douglas, for their help in our clinical studies. Finally, I thank heaven for Mary Jo Boya, her editing skills, and her unprecedented generosity.

—S.B.

I acknowledge and am grateful for the many leaders in the field of holistic health care whom it has been my good fortune to meet and work with over the years. As always, I'd also like to thank my parents, siblings, nieces, nephews, and friends for their ongoing love and support. Additionally, I acknowledge and thank Dr. Susan Brown, without whom this book would not have been possible.

—L.T.

Together, we would like to acknowledge our debt to the many scientists, researchers, and health practitioners, past and present, who have dedicated themselves to furthering our understanding of the importance of acid-alkaline balance for good health. Without their contributions, this book could not have been written. However, while we acknowledge and deeply appreciate their work, we are solely responsible for the perspectives, data, and estimations of the relative acid-forming or alkaline-forming impact of foods presented in this book.

Finally, we would like to thank our publisher, Rudy Shur, who conceived of this project and guided us every step of the way to its completion. Thanks, too, to Rudy's staff at Square One Publishers, who always go the extra mile in all that they do.

INTRODUCTION

The importance of diet has been a basic tenet of traditional healing systems around the world for many centuries. A wholesome diet not only helps to maintain health, but can also play a vital role in recovery from disease. On the other hand, it is safe to say that unhealthy dietary patterns are a major contributing factor in most disease conditions. Although for many years mainstream medicine ignored the role that diet can play in both health and disease, more recently it, too, began emphasizing the need to eat wisely and healthfully as a primary self-care approach for keeping illness at bay. For example, whereas only a few decades ago the American Cancer Society and the American Heart Association made little mention of the link between cancer, heart disease, and diet, today both organizations recommend the daily consumption of at least five to seven servings of fresh fruits and vegetables. Moreover, the American Cancer Society now states that as many as a third of all cases of cancer in the United States could be avoided if we as a nation adopted healthier eating habits.

The wisdom behind such recommendations is well known to pet owners. Whenever a beloved animal becomes sick, the veterinarian typically recommends a change in the pet's diet. Often, this alone is enough to reverse the problem or, at the very least, improve the pet's symptoms. Nutritionally oriented physicians have for many years reported similar positive results when their patients make positive changes in their own diet.

Our understanding of how and why certain foods can significantly help to improve health, while other foods can accelerate the disease process, continues to grow each year as scientists continue their quest to uncover Nature's secrets. In recent years, one of the most exciting nutritional discoveries has concerned the effect that different foods have on the body's pH levels once they are consumed. Simply put, some foods, once digested, create an acidic effect within the body, while others act as alkalizing agents that can neutralize harmful acids. To be healthy, it is necessary to be in a state of acid-alkaline balance. Humans have, in fact, a genetically encoded requirement for a dietary balance of acid-forming and alkaline-forming foods. Because of our early ancestors' abundant intake of fruits, vegetables, nuts, and seeds, we evolved on diets high in organic mineral compounds—particularly potassium, magnesium, and calcium. We still need these compounds in order to maintain our internal acid-alkaline (acid-base) balance. But as you will discover, contemporary eating patterns are at odds with our ancient biological machinery, much to the detriment of our health.

It has been rightly said that both health and disease begin in the cells, for it is at the cellular level that the vast majority of the body's multitude of interactions occur. For example, in order for the body's cells to function properly, they need to receive life-giving nutrients and oxygen from the bloodstream, and at the same time, they need to release cellular wastes. As it turns out, both of these interactions can optimally take place only when the body is in a slightly alkaline state, which allows for an easy flow of oxygen and nutrients into the cell walls and an equally easy disposal of cellular waste. When the body becomes chronically acidic, however, these and many other cellular processes start to become impaired. Eventually, if acidity continues unchecked, the combination of a diminished oxygen and nutrient supply to the cells and the buildup of wastes inside the cells sets into motion both fatigue and disease.

It's precisely for this reason that both the American Cancer Society and the American Heart Association—along with the American Medical Association and most other health organizations—recommend a minimum of five servings of fruits and vegetables each day. Why are fruits and vegetables so important? Because, as suggested above, most fruits and vegetables are high in compounds that help to keep your body in the slightly alkaline state that medical research has shown is the ideal internal environment for achieving and maintaining optimal health.

As you will learn in the chapters ahead, the importance of maintaining proper acid-alkaline balance is not a new concept. In fact, it has been written about in medical textbooks for more than a century. Only in the last few years, however, has the concept of chronic, low-grade acidosis started to make its way to the public at large, primarily through infomercials and certain books. Unfortunately, such information is all too often tied into products for which dubious claims are made, or associated with dietary plans that are too restrictive for most people. But at this same time, a small number of brilliant scientists from around the world have recognized, and are studying, the phenomenon of chronic, low-grade metabolic acidosis. Scientists such as Dr. Lynda Frassetto at the University of California, San Francisco, and Dr. Russell Jaffe of ELISA / ACT Biotechnologies, Inc., have documented that on the whole, the average Western diet is acid-producing, and that it actually produces a low-grade systemic acidosis in otherwise healthy people. Dozens of such studies further document the negative impact that low-grade acidosis has on health. Osteoporosis, age-related muscle loss, kidney stone formation, gout and other joint diseases, and back pain are among the conditions associated with the move towards an even *slightly* acidic state. While not life threatening, this low-level acid condition compromises our health.

Today in the United States and other highly Westernized countries, chronic low-grade acidosis is more the rule than the exception. This is largely due to poor eating and lifestyle habits. We are, in fact, forcing our bodies to labor within a less-than-optimal biochemical environment. The body's adaptation to even mild metabolic acidosis involves stresses and strains that create a fertile breeding ground for the various forms of chronic illness that are now experienced by more than one out of every three Americans.

Since your diet dramatically affects acid-alkaline balance either positively or negatively, you might ask yourself how you can change any unhealthy eating habits in a safe and practical manner—without having to make drastic changes. *The Acid-Alkaline Food Guide* was written precisely to answer that question. In the pages that follow, you will find listings of literally hundreds of our most commonly eaten foods and be able to quickly determine how they will affect your body's pH levels once they are consumed and digested. And once you know the effects that these foods will have on your body, you will be able to quickly and effectively create healthy meal plans using the foods you already enjoy.

The Acid-Alkaline Food Guide is the first and only book of its kind to provide this information in such extensive detail. Moreover, the information that it contains is based on hard science—on research conducted specifically to determine the effects that various foods have on the body's acid-alkaline balance. In this book, you will discover:

❏ What a pH and an acid-alkaline balance are, and why they are so important to your health.

❏ How an acid-alkaline imbalance encourages the development of disease.

❏ Which health disorders are associated with a state of acid-alkaline imbalance.

❏ How to measure your own acid-alkaline balance.

❏ How to quickly determine whether a food will produce an acidifying or alkalizing effect on your body.

❏ How to use the food tables presented in this book to create healthy meals throughout the day.

❏ How to use nutritional supplements to speed your journey to vibrant health.

More than 2,500 years ago, the Greek physician Hippocrates said that food should be our first and most important "medicine." Here in the twenty-first century, the truth of that adage has never been clearer. It is our hope that *The Acid-Alkaline Food Guide* will empower you to make wise food choices that result in good health and vitality for both you and your loved ones.

PART ONE

UNDERSTANDING
ACID-ALKALINE
BALANCE

1. ACID-ALKALINE BALANCE FOR GOOD HEALTH

When it comes to health, balance is everything. Specifically, to ensure good health, the body needs to maintain the proper balance between two basic types of chemical compounds—acids and alkalis. The balance of these compounds is essential for both minute-to-minute and long-term survival, and creates what is known as the pH value of our body's fluids, which include blood, saliva, urine, and the fluids both between and inside the cells.

Albert Szent-Gyögyi, Nobel Laureate and the discoverer of vitamin C, once noted, "The body is alkaline by design, but acidic by function." He was referring to the fact that each minute of each day, the body's metabolic processes produce enormous quantities of acid even though, in order to do their jobs properly, the cells and tissues require a slightly alkaline environment. Therefore, in order to maintain its health, the body must neutralize or excrete the vast majority of acids that it produces on a minute-to- minute basis. Healthy bodies maintain a narrow range of pH blood and tissue balance at all times. For this reason, proper acid-alkaline balance is one of the most essential elements of optimal health, while imbalances between acid and alkaline compounds are certain signs that the body is in danger of becoming unhealthy and increasingly susceptible to disease.

In this chapter, you will learn what pH actually means and why balanced pH body chemistry is essential for optimum health. You will also see the various mechanisms used by the body to maintain a healthy pH. Finally, you will be introduced to the new scientific concept of chronic low-grade metabolic acidosis, which is at the heart of many negative health conditions.

WHAT pH IS AND WHAT IT MEANS TO OUR HEALTH

The term pH was originally defined in 1909 by Søren Peter Lauritz Sørensen, a Danish biochemist. Literally meaning "potential for hydrogen," pH is used to indicate the concentration of hydrogen ions in a fluid. Since dissolved acids are what produce hydrogen ions, we know that the more hydrogen ions there are present, the more acidic the solution will be. Therefore, by showing the concentration of hydrogen ions, pH also indicates whether a fluid or compound is acidic, alkaline, or neutral. That's why the measurement of pH in our fluids and tissues allows us to determine whether our bodies are in a state of acid-alkaline balance. (For more information on pH and hydrogen ions, see the inset on page 12.)

pH is measured on a scale of 0 to 14. A measurement of 7 is neutral; in other words, it is neither acidic nor alkaline. Any measurement lower than 7 is considered acidic, and any measurement higher than 7 is considered alkaline. As concentrations of hydrogen ions increase in a substance, so does the acidic level.

Since the time when pH measurements were first used, medical researchers have shown that in order for the body to remain healthy, a slightly alkaline, oxygen-rich arterial blood pH reading of 7.365 to 7.45 is necessary. A significant shift away from these ideal pH values is not compatible with life, and will therefore cause death within a short period of time. In this book, we are concerned with much smaller—and more common—diet-induced movements away from ideal blood pH. Although these relatively small shifts in acid-base balance are not immediately life threatening, they nevertheless endanger our health in subtle ways and help set the stage for the development of disease.

The link between pH balance and disease has been recognized by physicians since the early twentieth century, and today, every medical physiology textbook discusses the extreme life-threatening forms of acid-base imbalance. For instance, Arthur C. Guyton's *Textbook of Medical Physiology*, an essential reference in medical schools, states, "The regulation of hydrogen ion concentration is

The Relationship Between pH and Hydrogen Ions Within the Body

As explained on page 10, the pH or acid-base status of a substance is determined by the substance's concentration of hydrogen ions, which are simple protons (positively charged particles). By definition, an *acid* is a substance that gives off hydrogen ions, while its opposite, a *base* (also known as an *alkali*), is a substance that accepts hydrogen ions.

All acids in the body contain hydrogen ions in varying concentrations, with stronger acids having a greater concentration of hydrogen ions than weaker acids. The hydrogen ion is unstable and very reactive. Specifically, it seeks to react with a negatively charged molecule. So hydrogen ions can be thought of as "hiding" in the body's water molecules, ready to react with other molecules. These hydrogen ions, once they become attached to various proteins, alter a protein's structure, or "denature" it. This is precisely how hydrochloric acid in the stomach aids in protein digestion.

Because an acid gives off hydrogen ions while a base accepts hydrogen ions, acids and bases can react with one another, altering the acid-base balance of a substance. In the body, the bicarbonate ion is a major base that transforms and neutralizes acids by taking on their hydrogen ions. Largely, it is the balance between bicarbonate and hydrogen ions that determines acid-base balance.

It is worth noting that pH values are determined by the concentration of hydrogen ions represented as moles per liter. (The term *mole* is short for *molecular weight*.) Pure water, which is a neutral element, has a concentration of hydrogen ions that equals 0.0000001, or 10^{-7} moles per liter. By comparison, extremely acidic substances can have hydrogen ion concentrations as high as 0.01, or 10^{-2} moles per liter. As these examples make clear, the concentration of hydrogen ions in a substance is written as a power of 10. To indicate the substance's pH value, we remove the base number 10 and the minus sign. Thus, a pH of 7 is the value of pure (neutral) water, while a pH of 2 indicates very high acidity, and a pH of 12 indicates very high alkalinity. An increase of one point of pH is equal to a ten-fold decrease in hydrogen ion concentration, while a decrease of one point of pH equals a ten-fold increase in hydrogen ion concentration.

one of the most important aspects of homeostasis." In other words, the body's pH must be regulated if the body is to maintain a stable internal environment that permits proper functioning of its component cells, tissues, organs, and organ systems.

Despite this understanding of the importance of pH in the maintenance of life, until recently, the mainstream medical establishment overlooked the existence of low-grade pH imbalances. Fortunately, for decades, holistic physicians both in the United

States and in Europe have recognized the link between chronic low-grade acid-alkali imbalance and disease. In fact, in 2000, German pH researcher Dr. Jurgen Vormann organized a scientific conference entitled Acid-Base Metabolism: Nutrition-Health-Disease, at which researchers from around the world documented the impact of low-grade metabolic acidosis on health issues as diverse as bone health and growth in early childhood. As this information is shared and further research is performed, a greater appreciation of the pH-health connection is sure to become more common.

Are health problems ever caused by an overly *alkaline* body environment? Although a small number of people who are ill might have pH levels that are excessively alkaline, the vast majority of people experiencing less-than-optimal health or overt illness have pH levels that are overly acidic. As mentioned earlier, scientists identify this common, mildly acidic tilt in body chemistry as *chronic low-grade metabolic acidosis*. The primary force creating this low-level acidosis is our diet. The typical Western diet is *acidogenic,* meaning that it consists primarily of foods that have an ongoing acidifying effect on the body. This is especially true of the so-called standard American diet, which health experts now recognize as one of the leading causes of our nation's rising rate of chronic, degenerative diseases, as well as a leading cause of the epidemic of obesity that is now occurring among our country's children.

Given that acid-alkaline balance is essential for your survival, your body gives top priority to its maintenance. The next section examines how various mechanisms work to maintain a healthy pH within the body.

HOW THE BODY MAINTAINS ACID-ALKALINE BALANCE

Various multi-layered physiological mechanisms act to ensure that the pH values of the cells, fluids, tissues, and organs are properly maintained. They do so by neutralizing and eliminating excess acid buildup. What follows is a simplified overview of how these mechanisms function.

First, there are several layered buffer systems within the cells and the blood that work to neutralize or buffer acid by-products. These buffer systems—known as the bicarbonate, phosphate, and protein buffer systems—help maintain stable cellular and blood acid-alkaline balance.

The primary organs that work to eliminate acid buildup in the body are the kidneys and the lungs, followed, to a lesser extent, by the skin. Although some of these organs play a more significant role than others, they are all engaged in the important activity of preserving internal pH balance.

The kidneys help regulate acid-alkaline balance of the bloodstream by eliminating *solid acids*, also known as *fixed acids*—especially sulfuric and uric acid—through urination. When the levels of such acids become excessive, the kidneys excrete increased levels of hydrogen ions. This process acts as a filtering mechanism that dilutes the acids and moves them out of the bloodstream to be eliminated by the urine. In its excretion of acids, the kidneys utilize various alkali reserve compounds, and if these are not available from the diet, the body calls upon alkali reserves stored in the watery layer around the bone and in the bone itself. At times, even the muscles are affected as muscle tissue is broken down to release an alkalizing amino acid called glutamine, which is used by the body in its pH recovery-rescue processes.

Details of the complicated processes by which the kidneys eliminate acids from the body are beyond the scope of this book. However, it is important to note that through the use of bicarbonate and other alkalizing compounds, the kidneys are able to accomplish their task of neutralizing and removing acids as long as proper acid-alkaline balance is maintained. Note that the acids *must* be buffered with alkalizing compounds prior to their elimination, because without buffering, harsh concentrated acids with a pH of 4.5 or less would burn the delicate kidney tissues.

Regardless of how hard the kidneys work, or how efficient they are at producing and recycling alkalizing bicarbonate, these organs can rid the body of only a certain amount of acids each day. If the alkali reserves necessary for neutralizing acids are in short supply, while at the same time the body's production of acids is high, a degree of *aci-*

dosis, or acid buildup, occurs within the body. This buildup of acids beyond the kidneys' capacity to eliminate them can set the stage for a wide variety of health problems, beginning with the disruption of proper cell function. Then, over time, numerous biochemical reactions are impaired and the stage is set for dysfunction and disease.

The lungs also work to keep the body's pH levels balanced by eliminating volatile (gas-formed) acids. As you breathe, the carbon dioxide produced through metabolic processes inside the body combines with water in the blood. This combination produces carbonic acid, which the lungs then eliminate as part of the process of respiration, helping to keep overall acidity in check. One telltale sign that the body is becoming overly acidic is increased respiratory rate. This increase is caused by the body's attempts to eliminate increased levels of carbonic acid. Conversely, if the body is overly alkaline—a condition known as *alkalosis*—the rate of breathing generally decreases. This is because the body is attempting to retain enough acids to reverse excess alkalinity and restore proper acid-alkaline balance. In the average individual, the production, neutralization, and excretion of gaseous volatile acids goes on unaffected by dietary practices. Just as important, this process generally does not add an acid load to the body.

The skin, through its sweat glands, is the final organ responsible for eliminating acids. The skin accomplishes this through perspiration, which helps to flush acids out of the body. However, the amount of acids the skin can eliminate is not as significant as the amount eliminated by the kidneys and lungs. The body is capable of eliminating an average of only one quart of sweat every twenty-four hours, whereas it can eliminate one and a half quarts of urine. Moreover, sweat is unable to eliminate acids in the same concentrations that urine can. It is interesting to note that, since increased levels of acids contained in sweat can produce a strong smell, body odor produced by perspiration can be a strong indication of a state of over-acidity.

UNDERSTANDING THE SIGNIFICANCE OF BODY pH

Many people find it hard to believe that even relatively small fluctuations of the body's pH can have a profound impact on their health. A simple analogy can help to clarify the significance of these fluctuations.

Consider normal body temperature, which for most people is 98.6 degrees Fahrenheit. Should your body temperature fall below or rise above 98.6 degrees for any length of time, you start to feel unwell. In fact, even a modest variation in body temperature—one degree, for instance—causes distress and unease, while an extreme variation can lead to permanent damage or death. Although we may not be able to immediately sense the consequences of small fluctuations in body pH, the consequences are very real.

People also question the long-term effects of acidosis on the body. This time, think of the environmental problems associated with acid rain, which has been shown not only to increase the acidity of water to the point where fish and other aquatic life can no longer survive, but also to cause adverse soil conditions and, ultimately, harm the health of plants. One of the primary causes of acid rain is the excess production of carbon dioxide, which is released into the atmosphere as a result of fossil fuel combustion as well as various industrial processes. In recent years, scientists have discovered that the earth's oceans act as enormous "acid sinks," helping to neutralize atmospheric carbon dioxide, an acid, with their calcium carbonate. Unfortunately, this process is leading to the demineralization and acidification of the oceans—a condition that contributes to environmental problems such as global warming, shifting weather patterns, and other ecological concerns.

Just as acid rain removes calcium carbonates from the ocean, a buildup of acidity within the body results in a loss of the mineral compounds used by the body to buffer metabolic acids. Just as our planet is undergoing the process of demineralization of its soils and waters due to the acid products of fossil fuel consumption, we are suffering the demineralization of our bodies due to our dietary practices. And as you will see in the next chapter, the burden of this demineralization could well be felt by every cell in the body.

CONCLUSION

You should now have a better understanding of what pH is, and of how the body works to maintain an ideal acid-alkaline balance. With this understanding, let's move on to explore the various unhealthy consequences of abnormal acid-alkaline levels. In the next chapter, we will examine the specific ways in which chronic low-grade metabolic acidosis interferes with the body's self-healing mechanisms, and we will explore the adverse health conditions that occur as a result.

2. THE CONSEQUENCES OF ACID-ALKALINE IMBALANCE

As you learned in Chapter 1, chronic acid-alkaline imbalances lead to one of two states—*alkalosis*, a condition characterized by excessive alkalinity in the body, or *acidosis*, a condition characterized by excessive acidity. Extreme imbalances in either direction are life threatening, but are relatively uncommon. However, even low levels of either condition can cause serious health problems if acid-alkaline balance is not restored.

Of the two states, acidosis, particularly chronic low-grade metabolic acidosis, is by far the most common acid-base imbalance affecting people in the United States and other Westernized nations. In fact, in these cultures, low-grade acidosis is more the rule than the exception. That is why this chapter first explores in detail the many health problems that can and often do result from persistent over-acidity. It then takes a brief look at the less-common form of pH imbalance—over-alkalinity.

CHRONIC LOW-GRADE ACIDOSIS

As you now know, by far the most common form of acid-alkaline imbalance, chronic low-grade metabolic acidosis is caused by a persistent buildup of excess metabolic acids within the body. This process tends to occur with age as kidneys weaken, but can be created in even the very young by our dietary patterns. These dietary patterns involve the overconsumption of acid-forming foods—such as proteins, grains, sugar, refined foods, coffee, and alcohol—and the underconsumption of alkaline-forming fruits, vegetables, nuts, and seeds. As a result of these patterns, our biochemistry labors under a slight yet chronic acid tilt that produces a fertile breeding ground for a variety of health problems.

How Chronic Low-Grade Metabolic Acidosis Harms the Body

As you have come to understand, the body constantly works to maintain ideal acid-base balance. When factors such as the intake of acid-producing foods makes the body chemistry more acidic, the body—from the cells to the kidneys to the skin—works quickly to compensate for this metabolic acidosis. But while these efforts to balance pH are essential, they are not without their own negative side effects. In essence, this pH balancing act leads to a depletion of alkali mineral reserves from the body, which, in turn, has many health implications.

A number of scientific studies have illuminated the "biological costs" of our forced adaptation to chronic acidosis. The problems caused by this condition include the following:

❑ Loss of calcium in the urine, the dissolution of bone, and the development of osteoporosis.

❑ Reduced bone formation.

❑ Increased levels of blood parathyroid hormone, a hormone that can cause bones to become brittle and prone to fracture.

❑ The loss of potassium and magnesium stores from the body, with a resulting tendency towards hypertension (high blood pressure) and inflammation, as well as the pain associated with inflammation.

❑ Protein catabolism (the breakdown of protein), resulting in muscle wasting and the worsening of age-related loss of muscle mass.

❑ Depressed protein metabolism, resulting in the inability to fully repair cells, tissues, and organs.

❑ Irritation of the urinary tract and bladder that, coupled with poor tissue repair, can lead to frequent and painful urination.

❑ Suppression of growth hormone, insulin-like growth factor, and other pituitary hormones, causing suboptimal tissue renewal and hormone dysfunction.

❑ Accelerated aging from accumulated acid waste products.

❑ Increased production of *free radicals*—unstable molecules that cause cellular damage—resulting in the worsening of pain and inflammation, and the lowering of immune capacity.

❑ Greater oxidation of free radicals and impaired activity of *antioxidants*—substances that protect the body from free radical damage—increasing the risk of degenerative disease and premature aging.

❑ Tendency for connective tissue to weaken due to increased free radicals generated by chronic inflammation, leading to further inflammation and pain.

❑ Increased risk of kidney stone formation.

❑ Decreased efficiency of cellular ATP energy production, causing impaired cellular function and, eventually, impaired organ function.

❑ Increased fluid retention, resulting in the excessive accumulation of fluids within body tissues.

❑ Disrupted balance of intestinal bacteria, with related digestive problems.

❑ Encouragement of the growth and spread of naturally occurring yeast and fungi, which thrive in an acid terrain.

❑ More fertile breeding grounds for many viruses, including HIV, which require an acidic environment combined with a low level of disease-fighting antioxidants.

❏ Reduced size of the brain's pool of energy reserves, causing weakened mental capacity.

❏ Decreased ability to perform exercise at a high level of intensity.

❏ Increased acidity of the mouth, leading to imbalanced oral bacteria and, consequently, increased dental decay and periodontal (gum) disease.

❏ Creation of a mild form of hypothyroidism (low thyroid function) and a chronic overproduction of the stress hormone cortisol, resulting in various negative effects on the body.

❏ Development of low blood phosphorus levels, which can result in loss of appetite, anemia, muscle weakness, and other health problems.

❏ Suboptimal liver detoxification, potentially causing a buildup of toxic residues in the body.

The above "laundry list" of acidosis-related problems shows just how damaging acid-alkaline imbalance can be to the body. In the following pages, we'll take a closer look at some of these problems so that you will have a greater understanding of how acidosis can cause and contribute to a variety of common health disorders.

Impaired Cellular Function

Much of the damage caused by an acid-alkaline imbalance occurs within the body's cells. All cells, in order to function properly, need to be in a state of acid-alkaline balance. When they are not, their many functions start to become disrupted. This, in turn, not only causes disruptions in the tissues and organs that the cells are designed to serve, but can also significantly diminish the cells' ability to produce energy via the cellular "energy factories" known as mitochondria.

Located within the cells, mitochondria are responsible for producing a compound known as ATP (adenosine triphosphate), which furnishes the energy that cells, tissues, and organs require to function properly. Even a slight acidic tilt within the cells causes impaired function of mitochondrial electron transport, leading to both reduced energy production and increased energy consumption. Deficits of ATP caused by excessively acidic or alkaline pH result in fatigue, and can eventually cause pain and affect organ function.

To counteract the cellular problems caused by low-level acidosis, the body's mechanisms of *homeostasis*—its ability to self-regulate and thus maintain internal balance—call upon alkali mineral stores, such as the alkali salts of calcium, magnesium, and potassium. These minerals, which are stored primarily within the musculoskeletal system, are used by the body to quench acid buildup. If the fluctuations in acid-alkaline levels are only temporary, homeostasis is usually restored. But if the imbalances remain chronic and unaddressed, eventually the body's ability to maintain homeostasis is overwhelmed, leading to a state of "dis-ease" that will, over time, begin to attack the weakest and most susceptible organ systems. At a basic level, even low-grade acid-alkaline imbalance impairs the cells' ability to perform their duties efficiently.

Fatigue

As mentioned above, excess acid buildup inside the body creates an environment that impairs the ability of the mitochondria inside the cells to produce ATP, a compound that is essential for optimal energy production at the cellular level. This sets the stage for fatigue to occur. In fact, in her practice, Dr. Brown has found that the more acidic an individual's body becomes, the more fatigue he or she is likely to experience.

Compounding this problem is the fact that acidosis also diminishes the supply of oxygen available to the body's cells and tissues. Lack of oxygen further interferes with mitochondrial function, and also impairs the cells' ability to properly repair and replenish themselves.

The low-oxygen environment created by acidosis also promotes the growth of harmful microorganisms. (You'll learn more about this in the discussion of diminished immunity, found on page 28.) This, too, contributes to fatigue by interfering with the body's ability to properly assimilate and make use of the nutrients obtained from the foods you eat. The resulting nutritional deficiencies not only diminish the production of hormones and enzymes necessary for energy production, but can also adversely affect blood sugar levels, thereby reducing the body's normal levels of physical endurance. Moreover, as these harmful micro-organisms proliferate, they can disrupt the production of chemical compounds known as *electrolytes*, which serve as conductors of electricity within the body, further reducing the production and normal flow of energy in the body. Left unchecked, all of these factors can eventually result in a condition of chronic fatigue.

Diminished Immunity

The body's immune defense and repair mechanisms operate best in an exquisitely narrow pH range. Acid-alkaline imbalances can weaken the body's ability to ward off infectious microorganisms, such as bacteria, fungi, and viruses. The reasons for this are many, with two being of special importance to our discussion.

First, when blood pH becomes unbalanced, the cells of the body are unable to efficiently receive vital nutrients and oxygen from the blood supply. In addition, the cells start to experience difficulties in eliminating wastes. In both cases, these responses are caused by the decreased permeability of cellular membranes, now hardened by acid-alkaline imbalance. As the cell walls harden, not only are oxygen and nutrients unable to enter the cells, but waste products are unable to be excreted. Together, these factors lead to weakened cells that are no longer able to act as Nature intended.

The second factor that leads to diminished immunity concerns the way in which acid-alkaline imbalances make it possible for infectious agents to thrive and reproduce inside the body, as mentioned earlier. Contrary to popular opinion, we do not become sick simply from exposure to infectious pathogens. The truth is that we are all exposed daily to such microorganisms. In addition, literally tens of thousands of different types of potentially harmful bacteria live within our gastrointestinal tracts each and every day. Yet, for the most part, they are not, by themselves, able to cause illness. This is exemplified by the fact that during heightened times of infection, such as flu season, not everyone develops a cold or the flu, even though everyone is exposed to the viruses that cause them.

To a large extent, the factor that determines whether microorganisms cause illness is the pH of the body's internal environment. When the body maintains an acid-alkaline balance, the bloodstream is in an *aerobic* state—meaning that it is rich with oxygen. In this state, the body is able to defend itself against potentially harmful pathogens, as it has been found that pathogens cannot long thrive or survive in oxygen-rich environments. When acid-alkaline imbalances occur and become chronic, however, the bloodstream starts to become deficient in oxygen. This lowered oxygen status enables microorganisms that previously posed little health risk to become pathogenic (disease-causing), as the body is not able to effectively eliminate them.

Moreover, a low-oxygen environment is ideally suited for allowing such microorganisms to multiply quickly inside the body, making it increasingly difficult for the body's immune system to deal with them.

Inflammation

Another serious consequence of acidosis is inflammation. Inflammation is a natural bodily response to the need for repair, and is therefore essential to the healing process. Through the inflammatory process, worn-out tissue or tissue damaged by trauma or infection is broken down and recycled in preparation for its replacement with fresh vital tissue. But when inflammation or tissue breakdown becomes chronic, and the healing phase is not completed, a wide spectrum of potential health problems can arise.

Acidosis creates a fertile ground for inflammation in many ways. For example, the increased levels of harmful microorganisms caused by acidosis can lead to inflammation. (Think of how an infected finger becomes inflamed and swollen.) The corrosive nature of acids can also damage tissues and organs, causing inflammation. Acidosis also increases free radical production, which makes inflammation and pain worse, while again lowering immune capacity.

Furthermore, when tissues and organs are chronically exposed to excess acids, they begin to harden and/or develop lesions in order to protect themselves. As a further protective mechanism, they may start to swell in an effort to prevent acids from penetrating the tissues. Such inflammatory responses can occur anywhere in the body, but usually start in the organ systems that are weakest, as a result of genetics or pre-existing health conditions. If inflammation persists, it can eventually lead to a variety of disease conditions, including arthritis, bronchitis, colitis, neuritis (an affliction of the nerves), skin problems such as eczema and hives, and urinary tract disorders such as cystitis (bladder infection) and painful urination. In addition, chronic inflammation can lower immune function, which is already reduced due to the proliferation of unhealthy microorganisms.

Osteoporosis and Other Problems Related to Mineral Loss

As mentioned earlier, in order to help buffer excess acid buildup, it may become necessary for the body to draw upon its alkali mineral stores. The bones, of course, represent the body's largest storehouse of mineral reserves, but mineral stores can also be found in the teeth and various organs. Although occasional periods of mineral withdrawal from bones, teeth, and organs usually do not cause health problems, consistent mineral withdrawal, or demineralization—especially of calcium, magnesium, and potassium—can lead to serious disorders. One of the most common of these problems is osteoporosis, a condition of extreme bone fragility and increased low-trauma fracture risk. In fact, at this writing, some 10 million Americans over the age of fifty have osteoporosis, and an additional 34 million are at risk because of their low bone mass.

There is a clear link between osteoporosis and chronic low-grade metabolic acidosis. Around the world, the incidence of osteoporotic fractures varies by at least thirty-fold, with low-trauma fractures—the hallmark of osteoporosis—being rare in cultures that follow diets and lifestyle patterns conducive to proper acid-alkaline balance. A variety of population-based studies now document the association between a high intake of base-forming foodstuffs (mainly fruits and vegetables) and bone health. The beneficial effect of fruit and vegetable intake on bone mass is evident not only in premenopausal, perimenopausal, postmenopausal, and elderly women—those at greatest risk of osteoporosis—but also in growing girls and even men. Furthermore, a large cross-cultural survey indicated that those countries with the lowest incidence of hip fracture also have the lowest consumption of acid-producing animal protein, and, usually, a consumption of vegetable protein that exceeds their intake of animal products. Of course, the diets enjoyed by these cultures are very different from the typical Western diet, which is high in acid-forming animal proteins, and low in base-forming, pH-balancing foods.

Unfortunately, chronic bone mineral loss also contributes to other bone-related conditions, including rheumatism, osteoarthritis, and degeneration of the disks of the spine. Spinal degeneration, in turn, can result in other problems, such as chronic back pain and sciatica. Moreover, the long-term loss of minerals can diminish the health of teeth, making them more brittle, more sensitive to hot and cold foods, more prone to cavities, and more susceptible to chipping—problems that are common in Western countries, but rare in cultures with diets that promote acid-alkaline balance.

Chronic mineral loss can also affect the skin and nails. Lack of minerals often leads to dry skin that itches, cracks easily, and shows signs of premature aging. Mineral loss can also lead to brittle finger- and toenails that are prone to cracking and splitting. Other conditions commonly associated with chronic mineral loss include thinning hair and bleeding or overly sensitive gums.

Premature Aging and Accelerated Aging Muscle Loss

Another consequence of chronic low-grade metabolic acidosis is premature aging. This is due in part to the fact that even a slight tilt toward metabolic acidosis impairs cellular function—a condition discussed earlier in the chapter. (See page 25.) By impairing cellular function, acidosis prevents cells from properly producing and maintaining the proteins needed for cellular repair. And without the ability to repair themselves, cells age.

Aging is further accelerated by the fact that acidosis can weaken a body's organs, leaving them

Medication and the Body's pH

Most medications, whether prescription or over-the-counter, can upset the body's acid-alkaline balance, especially if they are used for a long period of time and taken in relatively large quantities. Those drugs that have an acidifying effect on the body include *antibiotics,* which are used to treat bacterial infections; *antihistamines,* which are used to reduce inflammation and combat allergies; *psychotropic drugs,* which are used to treat mental health problems; and *antiseptic drugs,* which are used to treat conditions such as urinary tract infections, as well as to prevent infection. Aspirin and all other nonsteroidal anti-inflammatory drugs (NSAIDS) are also acidifying, especially when taken in high doses. In fact, most medications have an acidifying effect on the body.

Do any drugs have an alkalizing effect? Some do. In fact, diuretics, which are used to reduce excess retention of fluids, and drugs that are used to treat heartburn can actually create a condition of *over*-alkalinity in the body. (For more information about antacids, see the inset on page 38.)

Certain drugs can also interfere with accurate pH readings, causing the readings to falsely indicate overly low or high pH levels. For example, ammonium chloride as found in some cold and cough medicines may produce acidic urine, while the glaucoma medicine acetazolamide may produce an alkaline urine. Conversely, imbalanced acid-alkaline levels can interfere with the effectiveness of some medications. For example, certain drugs used to treat urinary tract infections—such as streptomycin, neomycin, and kanamycin—are more effective when the urine is slightly alkaline, and less so when the urine is acidic.

We cannot here explore the full extent to which medications can affect pH balance, or urine pH can influence medication effectiveness. If you find it necessary to use a medication for more than a few days, it would make sense to discuss the issue of acid-alkaline balance with your physician.

less efficient. In addition, chronic acidity can diminish proper cognitive and mental function since acids negatively affect the brain's neurons. Recent German research further suggests that cerebral energy pools are lower in individuals with higher degrees of chronic metabolic acidosis. All of these factors contribute to the impaired mental acuity and memory problems that are often associated with aging.

An additional negative impact of even low-grade acidosis is the loss of muscle, parts of which are broken down to obtain the amino acid glutamine. The glutamine is then employed in the manufacture of ammonia, a base used to rescue the body from acidosis.

Problems With Enzyme Function

Enzymes are proteins that speed up chemical reactions within the body. Collectively, enzymes are responsible for every single activity that is performed by the body each day, from breathing, circulation, and digestion to immune and organ function, reproduction, movement, speech, and thought. Without enzymes, other vital substances in the body, including vitamins, minerals, and hormones, are unable to function properly. In addition, without a proper supply of enzymes, the body is unable to make use of proteins, carbohydrates, and fats in order to repair and rebuild itself. However, enzymes can perform their thousands of tasks only within a very narrow pH range.

In conditions of acid-alkaline imbalance, the body's enzymes start to malfunction. For example, Dr. Russell Jaffe estimates that there is a tenfold reduction in enzyme activity when the intracellular pH goes out of its normal range of 7.3 to 7.5 by even a tenth of one pH point. In some cases, enzyme activity can completely stop due to unhealthy pH levels. Both enzyme malfunction and the cessation of enzyme activity set the stage for disease. If proper acid-alkaline balance is not restored quickly, the ensuing disease can progress to a severe state. In the case of a complete halt of enzyme activity, even death can occur.

Although the malfunction of enzymes can be caused by both acidosis and alkalosis, typically, such problems are due to over-acidity.

ALKALOSIS

Although less common than acidosis, alkalosis, which is characterized by an excessively high alkaline state in the body, can also pose serious health risks. Diet rarely causes alkalosis, but the overuse of certain drugs has been known to contribute to over-alkalinity. Certain health conditions—and even certain environments—can also create a chronic alkali tilt within the body.

The drugs most often responsible for chronic alkalosis are the antacids used to treat and prevent heartburn. Such medications, when taken on a regular basis, can significantly disrupt acid-alkaline balance, leading to insufficient amounts of hydrochloric acid (HCl)—the acid used by the stomach to break down food. Drugs used to treat gastrointestinal ulcers and diuretics, which promote the elimination of body fluids, can also result in higher-than-normal alkaline pH levels. (For information on medications in general, see the inset on page 34. For information specifically on antacids, see the inset on page 38.)

Alkalosis can result from a variety of other conditions, as well. It can, for instance, be caused by chronic diarrhea or vomiting, both of which can reduce a body's levels of HCl and other acids. It can also be caused by a rare genetic predisposition to higher-than-normal alkaline pH levels. Overactivity of the adrenal glands can also contribute to alkalosis, as can anorexia nervosa—a psychophysiological eating disorder characterized by self-star-

Antacids

Antacids are used to relieve the symptoms of heartburn—one of the more common side effects of the highly acidifying standard American diet. Heartburn occurs when gastric acid backs up into the esophagus. Many people who suffer from regular bouts of heartburn use antacids such as Rolaids and Tums to deal with their symptoms. At best, these products offer only temporary symptom relief, but are not able to address the underlying causes of heartburn. Moreover, antacids contain strong alkalizing agents that neutralize the stomach's hydrochloric acid (HCl), and thus weaken digestion and interfere with the body's ability to absorb essential nutrients, including vitamin B_{12}, folic acid, and many of the minerals that help to buffer acid buildup. In addition, studies have shown that when antacids are used on a regular basis, they can actually worsen heartburn symptoms by disrupting healthy acid-alkaline balance.

vation and, in some cases, self-induced vomiting. Finally, people who live in high altitudes, where the oxygen content of the air is lower than normal, can be susceptible to alkalosis.

Chronic alkalosis can cause a range of health problems. Some, like fatigue, are relatively mild, but others are far more serious. The most common and serious health problem caused by chronic alka-

Ironically, most people who use antacids to treat heartburn mistakenly believe that their symptoms are due to an excess production of HCl. In reality, research published as far back as the 1960s in leading, peer-reviewed medical journals such as *Lancet* shows that many cases of heartburn are due to too *little* production of HCl, not too much. As HCl production decreases, some foods, especially those rich in proteins, may be only partially digested. This can lead to undigested food particles fermenting inside the stomach, causing heartburn and other digestive problems.

Fortunately, most cases of heartburn readily resolve themselves with dietary changes. These changes include avoiding any food to which you are sensitive or allergic; increasing the consumption of foods that have alkalizing effects; and, whenever possible, eating warm cooked foods, which are more easily digested than cold raw foods for most people who experience heartburn.

losis is hyper-excitability of the body's nervous system. Such heightened excitability affects both the *central nervous system*—the spinal cord and brain; and the *peripheral nerves*—the nerves that transmit messages from the spinal cord and brain to other parts of the body. When this condition occurs, initially the peripheral nerves start to automatically and repeatedly react even though they are not being stimulated. The end result is a painful condition known as *tetany*, which is characterized by cramps of the voluntary muscles, especially of the fingers, toes, and face. Alkalosis can represent a serious health condition not usually related to diet, and is best treated by a physician.

CONCLUSION

You should now have a greater understanding of the importance of acid-alkaline balance to your overall health. As you have learned, chronic pH imbalance can disrupt many body systems and lead to problems as diverse as impaired immunity, osteoporosis, and premature aging. How can you find out if your body has a balanced pH, or if it has a potentially harmful acidic tilt? In the next chapter, we will discuss simple means by which you can estimate your body's pH.

3. TESTING FOR pH BALANCE

If you have read Chapters 1 and 2, you are probably eager to know if your body is in a state of favorable acid-alkaline balance, or if you are experiencing some degree of acidosis. If you follow our nation's average contemporary diet, you most likely have some degree of chronic low-grade metabolic acidosis. But if your diet is high in nutrient-dense, mineral-rich foods, you may have a healthy pH balance.

It can be tricky to measure the body's acid-base balance. For one thing, different fluids in the body have different pH levels. Arterial blood has an average pH of 7.34 to 7.43, the pH of saliva can vary from 5.5 to 7.5 or more, gastric juices high in hydrochloric acid can have a pH of 2.5, and the pH of urine can fluctuate from 5 to 8 over the course of the day. In critical care medicine, doctors measure the pH of arterial blood, blood gases, and blood uric and lactic acid. But are any of these tests a good measure of chronic low-grade metabolic acidosis?

Because the kidneys are responsible for the handling of metabolic acids, the best test for low-level acidosis is a specific sample of urine—"specific" because, as mentioned above, urine pH varies during the day according to the foods consumed. (For more on this test, see the inset on page 43.) This is the test that Dr. Brown has been using for over a decade and a half to help her patients. In the following pages, you will learn how to use this simple test at home so that you can determine your own acid-alkaline balance.

MEASURING YOUR URINE pH

It is not difficult to estimate your metabolic pH. To do so, you will need two items: pH test paper, also known as Hydrion paper, and your own first-morning urine. Let's look at each of these items in turn.

Hydrion paper is a paper that has been impregnated with mixtures of indicator dyes. When this strip comes into contact with an acid or base substance, it changes color, with each color indicating a different pH value. The color of the paper is then compared with a color chart, and when a match is found, you know the approximate pH of the substance being tested.

To test the pH of your urine, you will want a pH paper that has small enough gradients to detect the 6.5-to-7.5 range. In her practice, Dr. Brown uses Hydrion paper that measures pH from 5.5 to 8 with twelve gradients in between—5.5, 5.8, 6.0, 6.2, and so forth. (For more about this special test paper, see page 183.)

Finding the Right Test

Earlier in the chapter, you learned that there are several methods of gauging the body's pH. Why, then, are we recommending that you test your first-morning urine?

This method of determining pH was developed by Russell Jaffe, MD, PhD, founder of ELISA/ACT Biotechnologies, and author of *The Joy of Food: The Alkaline Way Guide.* It has been used successfully by Dr. Jaffe and his colleagues for more than twenty years, and its validity was supported by research conducted at the University of Saskatchewan. Because it uses only the first-morning urine, this technique resolves the problem created by hour-to-hour variations in urine pH levels.

Another researcher—Dr. Ted Morter, author of *An Apple a Day*—developed a similar system for estimating acid-base balance from urine pH. Dr. Morter's testing system, however, involves the consumption of acid foods prior to testing. Dr. Brown has found that while that method is valid, it is more cumbersome than testing early-morning urine. In her work, she has used the early-morning urine test for a decade and a half, and has found it an easy and accurate way for patients to initially determine their acid-alkaline status, and then monitor their pH as they make healthy dietary changes.

As already mentioned, it is best to use first-morning urine to measure pH. Furthermore, the reading should be taken only after at least six hours of rest without urination. At that point, the kidneys will have done their night's work of buffering the acids, and the urine will not show the temporary effects of a meal or specific food.

To measure your pH, upon rising in the morning, simply wet the test paper with your urine, either by urinating directly on the test strip or by collecting urine in a cup and dipping the paper into the liquid. Then quickly place the wet paper on a tissue. Do not oversaturate the test paper by holding it in the urine for an extended period of time, as this may give you a false reading. The pH paper will take on a color immediately, and after five to ten seconds, you will be able to compare the color of the paper with the color chart that came with the test papers. (Do not wait longer than ten seconds or so to take the reading.) This will give you a fairly accurate indication of your body's pH.

In the beginning, we recommend that you test your first-morning urine as many days a week as possible. After a week or two, you will know your average baseline pH measurement. If you are acidic at baseline, like most people who eat a typical Western diet, you will be able to watch your pH level rise as you make appropriate dietary and supplement changes. This may take several weeks. Although you may not measure your first-morning urine every day after you've established a baseline, try to measure it often enough to have a sense of improvement.

INTERPRETING THE TEST RESULTS

Once you have used the test paper to determine your body's pH, how can you interpret the reading? As you might recall, a pH of 7 is neutral, any reading below 7 is acid, and any reading above 7 is alkaline. You now also know that the body functions best in a slightly alkaline state. Therefore, ideally you want your first-morning urine to have a pH between 6.5 and 7.5, with an occasional, but not regular, higher reading. This would indicate that your overall metabolic pH is mildly alkaline, and that the small amounts of acid that build up from normal metabolism are being excreted. (For a quick look at possible readings and their meaning, see the inset on page 47.)

If your pH reading is below 6.5, it is likely that you are experiencing an excessive acid load. This acid load is most probably caused by a diet high in acid-forming foods and low in base-forming foods. Don't be too upset. Dr. Brown has found this acid tilt to be the rule, while the individual with a more ideal pH is the exception. But if you come up with an acidic reading, you will want to begin making food choice changes aimed at alkalizing your diet. (You'll learn more about following a healthy diet in Chapter 4.) In most cases, this will result in a pH that slowly climbs to a more healthy range. If, however, you have a consistently low pH that does *not* respond to dietary changes or mineral supplementation, this could be a sign of a disease state that requires medical attention.

What if your urine pH reading is consistently very high—above 7.5 and approaching 8, for instance? Although uncommon, it is possible that this reflects a dangerous state of true over-alkalinity. (To learn more about this condition, see page 37 of Chapter 2.) Fortunately, though, most high urine pH readings do not reflect serious alkalosis, but instead indicate a *catabolic state*—a state in which the body is breaking down its own tissue. In this breakdown process, the amino acid glutamine, found in the muscles, is used to manufacture ammonia. As discussed in the previous chapter, ammonia is a strong base that helps the body rid itself of acids when other alkali reserves are depleted. In fact, ammonia alkalizes the urine to an even higher pH level than can normally be accomplished by alkali mineral salts. Therefore, a high false alkalinity reflects an underlying acidic condition that should, again, be treated with diet. And because cases of false alkalinity disguise a strong acid environment, it would be prudent to also consult with a health-care professional familiar with metabolic acidosis.

In reviewing your readings over time, keep in mind that even a small change in the numbers indicates a considerable shift in pH. As mentioned in Chapter 1, the move from one pH unit to another— from 6.5 to 7.5, for instance—shows a tenfold change in pH. So a pH of 7.5 is ten times more alkaline than a pH of 6.5.

WHAT IF YOU CAN'T SLEEP FOR SIX HOURS WITHOUT URINATING?

If you usually wake up during the night to urinate, and therefore don't get an uninterrupted night's sleep, first try making a modification in your rou-

---

A Quick Guide to Urine pH Readings

As discussed earlier in this chapter, the best time to test the pH of your urine is first thing in the morning, after a rest of at least six hours. It is best to test your urine several days in a row in order to get an accurate reading. Once you feel certain of your internal pH, the following table will help you quickly interpret the reading. (For a more complete discussion, see pages 45 to 47.)

TABLE 3.1. INTERPRETING YOUR pH READING

Your pH Reading	What It Means
Under 6.5	You probably have an acid condition.
6.5 to 7.5	You probably have an ideal acid-base balance.
Consistently 7.6 or higher	Although this can be an indication of alkalosis, it is more likely that this reading represents a "false alkalinity," and that you have an acid condition.

tine that will enable you to use the test once in a while—which should be adequate for the purpose of determining your pH. Try drinking less at night than you usually do, so that you sleep a longer period of time without waking. This may allow you to sleep for six hours at a stretch. And remember that it doesn't matter if you take the test in the middle of the night, as long as you haven't eaten or urinated for six hours. If you go to bed at 10:00 PM and wake to urinate at 4:00 AM, for instance, you'll be able to take your reading then and there, before returning to bed.

If you truly can't sleep for six hours without urinating, the urine test will not be useful for you. Fortunately, as an alternative, you can test your saliva. To perform the saliva test, you'll want to use the same Hydrion paper used for the urine test, and you'll want to perform the reading first thing in the morning, just as you would perform the urine test. Before you eat or drink, and before you brush your teeth, simply rinse your mouth a few times with water. Then, when you feel that you've generated some fresh saliva, dip the test strip in your saliva, place the paper on a tissue, and read it within ten seconds, comparing it with the color chart that came with the test paper.

Bear in mind that a saliva pH reading is often, but not always, a bit higher than urine pH. For example, a person with a 5.5 first-morning urine pH might have a slightly higher saliva pH. But, like the urine pH range, the acceptable range for first-morning saliva pH is 6.5 to 7.5, with a pH of about 7 being ideal.

CONCLUSION

Now that you know how to use pH strips to test for acid-alkaline imbalances, you can easily and regularly determine your body's pH level. If you find that your body is in a state of over-acidity, you're certainly not alone, because acidosis is an all-too-common symptom of our nation's standard diet of acidifying foods. Fortunately, there's a great deal you can do to correct this problem. The remaining chapters will show you how, by making a few simple changes in your diet, you can create an internal environment that's healthfully alkaline, and that minimizes the risks associated with chronic metabolic acidosis.

4. CREATING ACID-ALKALINE BALANCE

As you now know, your body's many functions, beginning at the cellular level, are performed most efficiently and effectively when your internal environment is in a state of acid-alkaline balance. Ideally, your body should be slightly alkaline, with an arterial blood pH reading of 7.35 to 7.45.

Because proper pH is essential for the performance of so many vital functions, your body has a built-in set of mechanisms that constantly work to maintain proper acid-alkaline levels. But as hard as it may try, the body cannot always achieve and preserve proper pH. When an individual consistently eats a diet that is largely acidifying—as is so often the case in Western countries—the body is forced to carry out its many functions in an unhealthy acid environment. All too often, the result of this situation is a variety of health disorders that, over time, can lead to the development of chronic degenerative disease.

Fortunately, there is much you can do to turn an unhealthy acidic environment into a health-promoting alkaline environment. In fact, the most important step you can take in creating an ideal acid-alkaline balance in your body is to take control of your diet by making smart food choices. This chapter will first look at how diet can create acid-alkaline imbalances, and then give you the direction you need to begin making simple dietary adjustments designed to optimize your long-term health.

HOW YOUR DIET CAN CREATE ACID-ALKALINE IMBALANCES

Whenever you eat food, it is metabolized, or broken down, for use in the body. Obviously, this process is highly complex, and a full explanation of it is beyond the scope of this book. But for the purpose of understanding body pH, all you really have to know is that while some foods end up contributing alkalizing bicarbonate to the body system, others end up producing acids. For example, the potassium citrate found in many fruits and vegetables is transformed through metabolism to potassium bicarbonate, which is a source of alkalizing bicarbonate. On the other hand, foods rich in sulfur-containing amino acids—high-protein foods such as red meat, poultry, and fish, as well as many grains and beans—are metabolized to produce a residue of sulfuric acid in the body. These foods are thus acid-forming.

Ideally, every meal that you eat should be composed of foods that contain a balance of alkalizing and acidifying substances. But for the majority of

Americans, this is not the case. Overall, the meals we eat are low in base-forming substances and high in acid-forming substances. Thus, the net impact of our eating patterns is to add an acid load to the body. In fact, research has found that most Americans suffer from a state of chronic low-grade acidosis that is directly related to the foods they most commonly consume. It is easy to understand why the nation is struggling with an ever-escalating health-care crisis.

When trying to appreciate how diet causes an unhealthy acid environment, it is vital to understand that the obvious chemical pH value of the foods you consume is not important. Rather, you have to know whether these foods end up adding to the body's alkali reserves, which can be used to neutralize acids, or contributing to free acids, which the body must then struggle to neutralize. Often, a food that most people think is acidifying has just the opposite effect once it is metabolized. For example, lemons and limes have a highly alkalizing effect, even though they are chemically acidic. This, in fact, is true for all citrus fruits, as well as some vinegars. What this means is that not all foods with inherently acidic pH values produce acidifying effects in the body when they are consumed. Nor are all inherently nonacidic foods alkalizing after they are metabolized. Chicken, for instance, certainly doesn't seem acidic, but when it is metabolized by the body, it has a moderately acidifying effect.

Unfortunately, physicians, nutritionists, and dieticians all too often ignore the issue of whether the foods they recommend promote or interfere with the body's acid-alkaline balance. Instead, they tend to focus on the nutrients provided by various foods—on protein, carbohydrates, fats, vitamins, and minerals, for instance. Certainly, nutrients play an important role in good health. Your body could not survive without the proper nutrients. But as explained in Chapter 2, your body is able to fully absorb and make use of nutrients only within specific pH levels. When your body enters a state of acid-alkaline imbalance, a number of problems result—ranging from the disruption of intestinal bacteria to impaired enzyme function—that interfere with the proper absorption and utilization of nutrients. If acid-alkaline imbalance persists, eventually nutritional deficiencies follow, and the stage is set for the progression of the disease process.

But the downward spiral just described doesn't have to occur. By following the guidelines presented in the remainder of this chapter, along with the food tables that begin on page 79, you will be able to make wise food choices that not only supply your body with the nutrients it needs, but also allow you to restore and maintain a healthy acid-alkaline balance.

CREATING A HEALTHY DIET

It is not difficult to follow a diet that promotes a healthy alkaline internal environment. As discussed earlier in the book, research indicates that during most of our vast evolution, the majority of the foods that humans consumed were base-forming. In Western societies, we've simply gotten into a lot of bad habits. But once we are armed with the proper information, we can break and re-form those habits and, in the process, greatly improve our health.

Choosing the Best Foods for Your Diet

The majority of foods you eat at every meal should be alkalizing. But your diet's precise proportion of acid-producing foods to alkali-producing foods should be determined by your internal pH level. In Chapter 3, you learned how easy it is to assess your body's pH. (See that chapter for details.) Once you learn your pH, you'll want to use that reading to guide your diet. And as you follow a healthier diet, you'll want to continue to monitor your acid-alkaline balance so that you can adjust your food choices as necessary.

In general, the more acidic your body's internal environment is, the greater number of alkalizing foods should be included in your diet. If your body's pH is slightly acidic to slightly alkaline—in other words, if it's in the healthful 6.5-to-7.5 range—60 to 65 percent of your foods should be alkaline-forming once digested. But if your body's pH level is either moderately acidic (6 to 6.4) or extremely acidic (5 to 5.9), 80 percent of each meal should be comprised of alkalizing foods. (For a fast overview of recommended acid-to-alkaline food ratios, see Table 4.1.) The higher your level of acidity, the longer you will probably have to stick to a diet high in alkalizing foods before your body is able to regain a healthy acid-base balance. Eventually, however, as your health improves and your body's pH swings away from acidity, you should be able to follow a diet comprised of only 60 to 65 percent of alkalizing foods, while continuing to maintain the health benefits you achieved.

TABLE 4.1. RECOMMENDED pH EATING PLANS

Your Urine pH Level	Recommended Percentage of Acidifying Foods	Recommended Percentage of Alkalizing Foods
Slightly Acidic to Slightly Alkaline (6.5 to 7.5)	35 % to 40%	60% to 65%
Moderately Acidic (6 to 6.4)	20%	80%
Extremely Acidic (5 to 5.9)	20%	80%

Which foods are most helpful in correcting an overly acidic internal environment? For the most part, you'll want to eat a good amount of fruits, vegetables, nuts, seeds, and spices, with green vegetables and root crops being especially helpful. By contrast, you'll want to minimize your consumption of acidifying foods such as meat, fish, poultry, milk, and dairy products. And you'll want to entirely avoid refined carbohydrates, refined sugar, coffee, sodas, and most highly processed foods, all of which are very acidifying. According to Dr. Russell Jaffe, the pioneering researcher first discussed in Chapter 3, if you are striving to correct an acid-alkaline imbalance, for every ten foods you eat, you should make six of them vegetables, with a special emphasis on leafy greens; two of them fruits; one of them protein; and one a high-starch alkalizing food, such as yams or potatoes.

Because a food's effect on the body is sometimes surprising, you'll want to refer often to The A-to-Z Listing of Basic Foods (see page 79)—especially when you first start to modify your diet. This listing presents a wide number of common foods and their acidifying or alkalizing effects. In some cases, you will find that although a food can be easily included in your new alkalizing diet, you have to make sure to choose the right form of that food. For instance, whereas natural sea salt is alkalizing in nature, commercial (processed) table salt is acidifying.

As you modify your diet to favor alkalizing foods, be sure to consider not only your overall food intake, but also each individual meal. Especially when trying to correct a problem of acidity, it is important to create meals that are predominantly alkalizing. Eating the bulk of your alkalizing foods during one or two meals and then eating acidifying foods the rest of the day will be far less effective. This is true of snacks, as well. By increasing your intake of alkalizing foods *every* time you eat, you will enable your body to more efficiently and effectively buffer the acids that are produced as your meals are digested and metabolized. Not only will this decrease the development of further over-acidity, but it will allow your body to more easily reduce and eliminate any acidic toxins that are already present.

Once you have fully restored your pH balance, you will probably find that you can occasionally indulge in an acidifying treat, such as pizza or ice cream, without causing problems. This is because over time, you will build up enough alkali mineral reserves to rescue your pH in times of overindulgence. Overall, however, the more consistent you are at eating a high proportion of alkalizing foods, even after you have improved your body's pH levels, the greater and longer-lasting your health benefits are likely to be.

Should You Eliminate Acidifying Foods From Your Diet?

Because eating a majority of alkalizing foods at every meal can significantly improve your acid-alkaline balance, you might consider it a good idea to *drastically* reduce the amount of acidifying foods you eat, or even to eliminate them entirely from your diet. But doing so would be a big mistake. Remember that even though high-protein foods such as meat, milk, and fish are acidifying, your body needs protein in order to build and repair tissues. Moderate amounts of protein, such as the RDA recommendation of 50 to 63 grams a day, are useful to the body. On the other hand, if you eat excessive amounts of protein, and especially if you fail to consume them along with alkalizing foods, you will add to your body's acid load.

Strangely, if you eliminate high-protein foods from your diet, you may be doing more than depriving yourself of essential nutrients. It seems that the body actually requires a certain amount of proteins each day in order to establish and maintain reserves of alkaline minerals in the cells and tissues. In their own way, blood proteins buffer acids, and a lack of sufficient protein hampers the neutralization of acids and is associated with eventual mineral loss.

In certain situations, a short-term diet composed solely of alkalizing foods may be warranted, such as in cases of severe acidosis accompanied by serious, painful symptoms. But even in these scenarios, a strictly alkalizing diet should not be followed for more than a few days, unless your physician advises you differently. Otherwise, you will deprive your body of needed proteins, as well as necessary vitamins, minerals, and essential fatty acids.

A Few Cautions to Keep in Mind

For most people, an alkalizing diet will, over time, promote good health and help avoid a variety of disorders. But sometimes, certain kidney disorders prevent individuals from neutralizing acids well. If you just can't seem to raise your pH to a healthful level despite dietary changes and the use of alkalizing supplements (see the inset on page 62 to learn about supplements), you should consider consulting your physician. Equally important, if you have kidney disease or if you use prescribed medications such as blood thinners, we recommend that you consult with your physician before making any significant change in your diet or using alkaline supplements.

Also remember that, although rare, some individuals do suffer from overalkalinity. (See page 37 of Chapter 2.) That's why it's important to follow the directions in Chapter 3 for assessing your body's pH. Then, if you suspect that you are suffering from a state of excess alkalinity, consider discussing this with your physician or other knowledgeable health-care professional.

Some Simple Tips for Healthy Eating

At this point, you should know the percentage of your diet that should be composed of alkalizing foods, and the percentage that should be made up of acidifying foods. You should also have a general idea of those foods that will help you alkalize your body, and those that will promote acidity. Over the years, though, Dr. Brown has found that when her clients first attempt to adjust their diet, they benefit from specific guidelines—from tips that make daily meal planning easier. By following the guidelines that begin on the next page, you will be able to more easily reverse the effects of over-acidity, bringing your body's pH levels closer to normal.

❏ In the morning, before breakfast, combine the juice of half a lemon or lime with eight ounces of water—preferably, spring water with a high mineral content. Repeat a few times during the rest of the day. As an alternative, substitute one or two tablespoons of organic apple cider vinegar for the fruit juice.

❏ Make lentils, as well as yams, sweet potatoes, and other root crops, staples in your meal plans. These foods help to quickly alkalize the body.

❏ Eat at least one cup of alkalizing green vegetables each day. Endive, kale, and collard, mustard, and turnip greens are especially healthful choices, as they are not only highly alkalizing, but also rich in important vitamins, minerals, and beneficial phyto-compounds.

❏ As often as possible, add alkalizing miso or seaweed to soups and other dishes. Also try adding a bit of grated ginger or daikon radish to your dishes. They will not only alkalize the dish, but will also spice it up and help to improve digestion.

❏ When eating grains, choose those that are more alkalizing. Excellent choices include organic oats, wild rice, and quinoa—a staple grain in South America that is increasingly found in our nation's health food stores and in the health food sections of many supermarket chains.

❏ Substitute alkalizing root crops—yams, turnips, sweet potatoes, rutabaga, jicama, burdock, lotus

The Benefits of Alkalizing Supplements

Although the focus of this book is on gaining and maintaining acid-alkaline balance through diet, some people are unable to achieve a healthy balance through diet alone. Sometimes, this is due to an inability to make sufficient dietary changes; sometimes, to an excessive depletion of minerals in the body; and sometimes, to extra-dietary factors such as stress. Whatever the reason, these individuals find that in addition to making alterations in the foods they eat, they need to use supplements that speed their return to health.

In her practice, Dr. Brown has found a variety of supplements to be helpful. For instance, many of her clients have achieved success through a mix of alkalizing magnesium salts—ionized magnesium glycinate, magnesium ascorbate, and magnesium citrate. Others have used a combination of alkalizing minerals and a specific form of vitamin C. And some have found it helpful to supplement with green vegetable drinks, which contain alkalizing greens such as barley and wheatgrass.

When choosing an alkalizing supplement, it is wise to avoid products that contain bicarbonate sources such as potassium bicarbonate or sodium bicarbonate (baking soda), which alkalize through the direct contribution of bicarbonate. Because the bicarbonate neutralizes hydrochloric acid (HCl), these supplements compromise digestion and thus reduce mineral absorption.

The list of alkalizing supplements that begins on page 177 will guide you to a number of effective products. Since these products come in different forms, ranging from easy-to-take capsules to drops and green drinks, you can choose the one that you feel best fits your lifestyle and your own preferences. Remember, though, that each person has a unique body chemistry, so that the supplement which works well for one person may not be right for another. Don't be afraid to try different supplements until you find the one that helps you achieve a healthful balance.

root, daikon radish, taro root, onion, kohlrabi, parsnips, and beets—for breads, pastas, flour, and other grain products.

❑ Eat several servings of fresh fruits a day, especially as snacks. Fruit salads are a great way to include a variety of nutrient-rich alkalizing foods in your diet.

❑ Drink spring water—especially one with a high mineral content.

❑ Consume fresh "green" vegetable juices, as they are great alkalizers.

❑ To further improve acid-alkaline balance, consider using alkalizing supplements. (See the inset above.)

CONCLUSION

Your daily food choices are among the most important factors affecting acid-alkaline balance. By following the general guidelines provided in this chapter, you can significantly improve your body's pH balance and, in doing so, improve your overall health and energy. However, the results you desire might take time to achieve, depending on how acidic your body's internal environment may be. Keep in mind that it probably took years for you to develop your current biological state, and that, depending on the degree of your mineral depletion, it may take several months to raise your pH level. Rather than being discouraged by this, be patient and persevere, because the long-term benefits to your health will be well worth the effort.

As you probably are aware, this book includes an A-to-Z Listing of Basic Foods—a comprehensive table of foods and their alkalizing or acidifying effects. (See page 79.) And for those people interested in food-on-the-go, it even includes a brief Fast Food Table. (See page 161.) How did we determine the pH-changing effects of all these common foods? That is the focus of the next chapter.

5. UNDERSTANDING THE FOOD TABLES

For decades now, health advocates interested in body chemistry have considered the effect of foods on the body's pH balance. If you have been interested in this topic for even a short time, you may have seen several different tables on the acidifying and alkalizing effects of foods. You might even have noticed discrepancies between the different tables. For instance, some tables categorize lemons as being acidic, while others describe them as being alkaline. This can be confusing and frustrating to the individual who is trying to adopt a healthy alkalizing diet.

The fact is that there are reasons for the differences between the tables—differences that often can be traced to the way in which people, over time, have arrived at their estimates of the effects of each food. This chapter will first take a brief look at the various methods that have been used to analyze foods, and then guide you in using the comprehensive food tables provided in this book to make the best selections possible for your health.

A BRIEF HISTORY OF pH FOOD ANALYSIS

Our understanding of different foods' acidifying and alkalizing effects has evolved over the years, along with the techniques for analyzing not only a food's composition before it is eaten, but also its composition after it has been metabolized by the body. Gradually, we have moved from "guesstimates" about the metabolic impact of foods to more scientific calculations. Let's look at a few of the steps that researchers have taken along the way.

From the early twentieth century until fairly recent times, estimates of acid-alkaline food impact were often based on the concept of acid and alkaline ash. The idea was simple. If you burned up a food and the ashes that remained contained "acid type mineral remains" such as sulfur, phosphorus, and iodine, the food was called acid-forming. On the other hand, if the ashes were of the alkaline type—if they contained calcium, magnesium, potassium, etc.—the food was considered alkaline-forming.

Over time, it became clear that the major issue was not the residue ash, but rather the types of chemical compounds the food contributed to the body *after* it was metabolized. The issue was the "metabolic effect" of the food—that is, the food's effect after it was processed by the body. Using this new concept, scientists began looking at the acid-base effects of individual food components, such as different minerals and amino acids. Once they knew the impact of each of these separate constituents, they began developing formulas to calculate the impact of a whole food. Given the complexity of human metabolism, this was a valiant task—one that scientists are now only beginning to perfect.

An excellent move toward quantifying the impact of foods on pH was made by two German scientists, Drs. Thomas Remer and Friedrich Manz. In 1995, they published their scientific formula for estimating the potential *kidney acid load* of foods—the amount of acid that ultimately reaches the kidneys for buffering and elimination. This new model was an elegant attempt to identify how foods affect urine pH and urine acid excretion, both of which indicate a food's effect on body pH. The model took into account the mineral and protein composition of foods, the average intestinal absorption rates of the respective nutrients, sulfur metabolism, and even urinary excretion of organic acids. Remer and Manz made the transition from looking simply at the chemical composition of a food to examining the broader after-digestion impact of its components. Their studies allowed them to produce a table showing estimates of the acid- or base-forming potential of numerous common foods.

Building on the work of Remer and Manz, Dr. Lynda Frassetto of the University of California looked again at the issue of food and its impact on urine acid excretion, and found that she could simplify matters. In 1998, Dr. Frassetto published her research findings, which indicated that kidney acid excretion could be estimated by an analysis of the protein-to-potassium ratio of the food consumed. In other words, she realized that by determining the amount of protein found in a food versus the amount of potassium, she could predict the amount of acid excreted by the kidneys, and therefore the amount of acid created by that particular food once it is metabolized. Specifically, she reported that 71 percent of the variation in kidney acid excretion could be accounted for by the ratio of protein (the major dietary acidifying force) to potassium (the major dietary alkalizing force).

While Dr. Frassetto developed an elegantly simple formula to estimate the influence of foods on acid excretion, Dr. Russell Jaffe developed a comprehensive, more complex formula for calculating the impact of foods on body pH. His formula includes not only the acid or alkaline contributions from all relevant minerals, amino acids (proteins), and organic acids, but also the influence of such food components as fatty acids, glycerides, and saccharides. Dr. Jaffe's more inclusive formula has been validated by his over twenty years of clinical experience reversing chronic low-grade metabolic acidosis.

The food tables that begin on page 79 present Dr. Susan Brown's estimation of the acid-forming or alkaline-forming nature of most common foods. Her categorization of foods as acid-forming or alkaline-forming is based on the scientific explorations of all the scholars listed above, combined with her own extensive clinical experience. In areas in which the above authorities offer conflicting conclusions, Dr. Brown has relied on the knowledge she gained working with hundreds of people as they adjusted their first-morning urine pH with dietary modifications.

The more we understand about our body's pH balance, the more we appreciate the complexity of our biochemical workings. Clearly, the tables presented in this book are a "work in progress," and over time, new scientific understandings will enable them to be refined and expanded. For now, these tables will provide you with a good basis for developing a life-supporting alkaline diet.

USING THE FOOD TABLES

You now know how over the years, scientists have developed different ways of making informed estimates of foods' acidifying and alkalizing effects on the body. Now it's time to look at the tables that will guide you in your food choices.

The tables that begin on page 79 of this book— the A-to-Z Listing of Basic Foods and the Fast Food Table—present the acidifying or alkalizing impact of a wide range of common foods, beverages, seasonings, and additives, and also list various popular combination foods, like pizza and macaroni and cheese. As you might expect, the A-to-Z Listing is comprehensive, and presents the data on both single foods and food combinations. The Fast Food Table, on the other hand, focuses on those items you're most likely to order in a fast food restaurant—hot dogs, hamburgers, tacos, French fries, and the like.

In addition to categorizing each food as acidifying or alkalizing, the tables also describe the *degree* to which each food is acid- or alkaline-forming. Tuna, for instance, is described as "Medium Acid-Forming," while lobster is "High Acid-Forming." This will allow you to choose the food from a category such as "Fish and Seafood" that will best help you meet the dietary goals you have established. Keep in mind, though, that the assignment of a "high," "medium," or "low" acid-forming or alkaline-forming classification was difficult at times. Understand, too, that the exact effect a food will have on *you* as an individual will depend on a number of factors, including your inherited genetic traits and unique biochemistry, the quality of the food, the methods used to grow and prepare the food, and any food allergies you may have. Therefore, while the calculations reflected in the tables are accurate for the vast majority of people, it makes sense to "go by results."

How can you "go by results"? First, pay attention to the way you feel following the consumption of each food. You may find that a food which has only mildly acidic effects on the general population affects you more severely, or that you have an allergy or hypersensitivity to an alkalizing food that, for most people, is quite healthful. In such a situation, you will want to avoid that food in the future. The second result you'll want to consider is the first-morning urine pH test detailed in Chapter 3. This is very important, because it assesses the effects of the foods you ate the previous day. As explained in Chapter 3, you'll want to keep your first-morning urine pH reading between 6.5 and 7.5. Initially, you'll probably find that in order to meet this goal, you have to cut down on acidifying foods or even avoid certain foods entirely. However, as your body builds more alkali mineral reserves, you should be able to increase your intake of acid-producing foods. You will then want to check your pH only occasionally to make sure that your mineral reserves are in place and that you are not slipping back into low-grade metabolic acidosis.

As discussed in Chapter 4, the food tables should be used to choose foods that fit into the eating plan determined by your pH. If your urine pH is only slightly acidic, for instance, you'll probably want to limit your intake of acidifying foods to about 35 percent of your diet, while if your pH is extremely acidic, only about 20 percent of your daily diet should be composed of acidifying foods. (See Table 4.1 on page 56.) In selecting the correct balance of acidifying and alkalizing foods, you will, of course, want to pay attention to the *amount* of each food you're eating. For instance, although paprika has been found to be highly alkaline-forming, sprinkling it over a highly acidifying steak will still result in a very acidifying meal. Your body might have enough alkali reserves, such as calcium, to buffer the acids created by the steak, but without

these reserves, you would have to consume per-
haps *four times* the amount of alkalizing foods, such
as salad greens, to compensate for the steak. The
point is that while alkalizing spices are good, you
should never fool yourself into thinking that they
will make up for an overall acidifying diet. Whenever you eat a food that is highly acid-forming, you
also must consume generous helpings of alkalizing
foods.

CONCLUSION

The food tables provided in this book are the result
of decades of research, analysis, and clinical experience. By using these tables to make informed food
selections, you will be able to first restore and then
maintain a healthy internal acid-alkaline balance.
Remember that the issue of pH balance is vital to
your overall health. By simply choosing to eat primarily alkalizing foods and following the dietary
guidelines provided in Chapter 4, you can dramatically reduce the amount of toxic acids your body
has to deal with in a safe and easy manner. In the
process, you will be creating better health and
increased energy, while at the same time avoiding
or alleviating a number of common health problems. It may take time before you fully realize the
benefits of a healthy pH balance, but with patience
and discipline, you will be able to enjoy greater
well-being than you may have experienced in years.

CONCLUSION

The importance of diet to health has been recognized by all of the world's healing traditions, from those of ancient China, Greece, and India, to those of modern-day Western cultures. As the acclaimed twelfth-century healer, philosopher, and rabbi Maimonides counseled, "No illness which can be treated by diet should be treated by any other means." Today, exciting research into the effects of foods on acid-alkaline balance provides a greater understanding of the wisdom behind such dietary advice. And now that you have read this book, it is our hope that you have a better appreciation of how the foods you eat can affect your body's acid-alkaline balance, and, by extension, your overall health.

With the information we have shared with you, especially the food tables, you now have the ability to improve your health simply by making smart food choices each and every day. Although the information presented here may be new and unfamiliar to you, you can prove its value to yourself simply by following the healthy eating guidelines we've provided and choosing wisely from the food and drink categories included in the food tables, which begin on page 79. Over time, as you become accustomed to this powerful new way of eating, the positive results will become increasingly clear. In addition you can, and should, gauge your results by using the urine pH test discussed in Chapter 3. Doing so will give you an objective measure of your progress as you move towards a more ideal acid-alkaline balance.

From time to time, you may find yourself craving acidifying foods, such as pizza and ice cream. Such impulses are only natural and if you find yourself succumbing to them, there is no need to get discouraged. Instead, simply make sure that the next few meals include highly alkalizing foods. Remember that it is how you nourish you body *most* of the time that is important, not the occasional "recreational" or "comfort" foods you consume. Also recall that the measurement of pH we discuss is really an indirect measure of mineral reserves. Given this, if you have a difficult time alkalizing with foods alone, you can use the various life-supporting alkali mineral supplements available today. (See the list on page 177.) What is most important is to be patient with yourself as you learn to incorporate new ways of eating and supplementing into your life as a means of achieving and maintaining proper acid-alkaline balance. The greater your commitment to this process, the easier it will become.

In closing, we would like to point out that the information provided in this book is by no means the final word. There is still a great deal to learn about food and its impact on acid-alkaline balance. Thus, although much has been discovered already, we look forward to updating this book as new information becomes available. In the meantime, we wish you optimum health, joy, and fulfillment.

PART TWO

THE FOOD TABLES

A-TO-Z LISTING
OF BASIC FOODS

The following table is a comprehensive list of foods, beverages, seasonings, and additives. As explained in Chapter 5, for each item listed, the table tells you whether the food is considered high, medium, or low alkaline-forming; or high, medium, or low acid-forming. (See page 70 for more information.) For the vast majority of foods, only one value—medium alkaline-forming, for instance—is given. Be aware, though, that in the case of a few sweetened foods, such as sweetened applesauce, the table shows a *range* of possibilities. This was done because while light sweetening may make a food only slightly more acidifying than its unsweetened version, a heavier use of sweeteners will have a more acidifying effect. You will want to keep this in mind both when you choose sweetened products and when you add your own sweeteners to foods. (For information on the alkalizing and acidifying effects of medications, see the insets on pages 34 and 38.)

A-TO-Z LISTING OF BASIC FOODS

FOOD	ALKALINE-FORMING			ACID-FORMING		
	High	Medium	Low	Low	Medium	High
Adzuki beans				■		
Agar seaweed *See also* Seaweed.		■				
ALCOHOLIC BEVERAGES						
Ale						
dark					■	
pale						■
Beer						
dark					■	
pale						■
Gin						■
Malt liquor						
dark					■	
pale						■
Scotch						■
Vodka						■
Wine						
red					■	
white					■	

FOOD	ALKALINE-FORMING			ACID-FORMING		
	High	Medium	Low	Low	Medium	High
Ale						
dark					■	
pale						■
Almond butter			■			
Almond milk (sweetened)			■			
Almond milk (unsweetened)			■			
Almonds			■			
Amaranth flour				■		
Amaranth seeds				■		
American cheese						■
Angel food cake						■
Apollinaris water *See also* Mineral water.	■					
Apple butter		■				
Apple cider		■				
Apple cider vinegar		■				
Apple crisp (with oatmeal and sucanat)			■			
Apple juice (sweetened)			■	■		
Apple juice (unsweetened)			■			
Apple pie (lightly sweetened) *See also* Pies, fruit.					■	

FOOD	ALKALINE-FORMING			ACID-FORMING		
	High	Medium	Low	Low	Medium	High
Apples						
baked (sweetened)		■				
baked (unsweetened)		■				
raw		■				
Applesauce (sweetened)		■				
Applesauce (unsweetened)		■				
Apricots		■				
Artichokes		■				
Artichokes, Jerusalem		■				
ARTIFICIAL SWEETENERS						
Aspartame					■	
Saccharin					■	
Asparagus	■					
Aspartame					■	
Avocado oil			■			
Avocados		■				
Bacon						■
Bagels, white flour *See also* Bread.						
cinnamon-raisin						■

FOOD	ALKALINE-FORMING			ACID-FORMING		
	High	Medium	Low	Low	Medium	High
egg						■
plain						■
water						■
Baked apples (sweetened)		■				
Baked apples (unsweetened)			■			
Baked beans (canned)						
with pork					■	
vegetarian				■		
Baked goods *See* Bread; Cakes; Cookies; Crackers.						
Baked potato, skin on, plain		■				
Baking chocolate *See also* Chocolate.						■
Baking powder	■					
Baking soda	■					
Balsamic vinegar				■		
Bananas		■				
Barley, whole grain					■	
Barley flour					■	
Basil		■				
Bass					■	
Bay leaf			■			

FOOD	ALKALINE-FORMING			ACID-FORMING		
	High	Medium	Low	Low	Medium	High
Bean sprouts *See also* Sprouts.		■				
Beans, baked (canned)						
with pork					■	
vegetarian				■		
BEANS AND LEGUMES						
Adzuki beans				■		
Baked. *See* Baked beans (canned)						
Black beans				■		
Chickpeas (garbanzo beans)				■		
Fava beans				■		
Great Northern beans				■		
Kidney beans				■		
Lentils		■				
Lima beans (butter beans)				■		
Mung beans				■		
Navy beans				■		
Peanuts					■	
Peas						
fresh green				■		
split peas, green and yellow				■		

FOOD	ALKALINE-FORMING			ACID-FORMING		
	High	Medium	Low	Low	Medium	High
Pinto beans				■		
Snow peas			■			
Soybeans						■
String, green, snap, wax, and yellow beans, *with* formed beans				■		
String, green, snap, wax, and yellow beans, *without* formed beans		■				
White beans				■		
Beef						
bologna						■
frankfurters						■
hamburgers						■
liver					■	
meat (steaks, roasts, etc.)						■
sausage						■
Beer						
dark					■	
pale						■
Beets		■				
Bell peppers						

FOOD	ALKALINE-FORMING			ACID-FORMING		
	High	Medium	Low	Low	Medium	High
green		■				
red		■				
yellow		■				
Benzoate (preservative)					■	
BERRIES						
Blackberries	■					
Blueberries		■				
Boysenberries		■				
Raspberries	■					
Strawberries	■					
Berry juice blend			■			
BEVERAGES						
Ale						
dark					■	
pale						■
Almond milk (sweetened)			■			
Almond milk (unsweetened)			■			
Apple cider		■				
Apple juice (sweetened)			■			

FOOD	ALKALINE-FORMING			ACID-FORMING		
	High	Medium	Low	Low	Medium	High
Apple juice (unsweetened)			■			
Beer						
dark					■	
pale						■
Berry juice blend			■			
Carrot juice				■		
Coffee (See inset on page 100.)						
decaffeinated (water decaffeinated)					■	
espresso						■
regular					■	
Cola drink (See page 142.)						■
Gin						■
Ginger tea	■					
Grape juice			■			
Grapefruit juice		■				
Malt liquor						
dark					■	
pale						■
Milk						
cow's milk, skim (nonfat)				■		

FOOD	ALKALINE-FORMING			ACID-FORMING		
	High	Medium	Low	Low	Medium	High
cow's milk, 1% fat				■		
cow's milk, 2% fat				■		
cow's milk, whole				■		
cow's milk, chocolate-flavored, whole					■	
goat's milk				■		
kefir (fermented cow's milk)					■	
rice milk					■	
soy milk						■
Milk shakes, commercial						
chocolate						■
vanilla						■
Orange juice			■			
Pear juice			■			
Pineapple juice		■				
Rice milk					■	
Root beer						■
Scotch						■
Soft drinks (carbonated), most types (See inset on page 142.)						■
Soy milk, most brands						■

FOOD	ALKALINE-FORMING			ACID-FORMING		
	High	Medium	Low	Low	Medium	High
Tea						
black tea, most types				■		
green tea, most types			■			
herbal tea, most types			■			
Tomato juice or juice blend				■		
Vegetable juice cocktail (commercial), tomato based			■			
Vegetable juice cocktail (homemade), green vegetables with apple, no tomato	■					
Vodka						■
Water, bottled mineral						
Apollinaris	■					
Evian			■			
Fiji			■			
San Pellegrino	■					
Sanfaustino	■					
Volvic			■			
Water, tap						
chlorinated, in general				■		
nonchlorinated, in general*				■		
Wine						

*Be aware that the value provided for nonchlorinated tap water is only an average, and that tap water can vary in its impact from region to region. See the inset on page 156 for more information.

FOOD	ALKALINE-FORMING			ACID-FORMING		
	High	Medium	Low	Low	Medium	High
red					■	
white					■	
Biscuits						■
Bison (buffalo)					■	
Black bean soup				■		
Black beans				■		
Black pepper		■				
Black tea, most types				■		
Blackberries	■					
Blueberries		■				
Bologna						
beef						■
bratwurst, link					■	
turkey					■	
Borscht		■				
Bottled water *See* Mineral water, bottled.						
Boysenberries		■				
Bran, oat					■	
Bran cereal					■	

FOOD	ALKALINE-FORMING High	Medium	Low	ACID-FORMING Low	Medium	High
Bran flakes and raisins (sweetened)				■		
Bran flakes and raisins (unsweetened)				■		
Bratwurst link bologna					■	
BREAD. *See also* Crackers.						
Bagels, white flour						
cinnamon-raisin						■
egg						■
plain						■
water						■
Biscuits						■
Breadsticks, white flour						■
Croissants						■
Matzoh						
white flour						■
whole wheat flour					■	
Pita						
white flour						■
whole wheat flour					■	
Pumpernickel					■	
Rye bread (100%)					■	

FOOD	ALKALINE-FORMING			ACID-FORMING		
	High	Medium	Low	Low	Medium	High
Tortillas						
corn					■	
white flour						■
White bread						■
Whole wheat bread					■	
Breadsticks, white flour						■
Breakfast sandwich with eggs, cheese, and sausage or ham						■
Broccoli		■				
Brown rice *See also* Rice.				■		
Brown rice cakes						
multigrain				■		
plain				■		
Brown rice flour				■		
Brown sugar *See also* Sugar.						■
Brownies *See also* Cake; Cookies.						■
Brussels sprouts			■			
Buckwheat flour				■		
Buckwheat groats (kasha)				■		

FOOD	ALKALINE-FORMING			ACID-FORMING		
	High	Medium	Low	Low	Medium	High
Buffalo (bison)					■	
Bulgur wheat (hard red winter)					■	
Burdock root	■					
Burgers *See* Hamburgers.						
Burritos						
with beef						■
with chicken						■
Butter				■		
Butter, clarified (ghee)			■			
Butter beans (lima beans)				■		
Cabbage						
Chinese		■				
red		■				
white		■				
Caesar salad dressing *See also* Salad dressings.						■
CAKES. *See also* **Desserts.**						
Angel food cake						■
Carrot cake, cream cheese frosting						■
Cheesecake						■
Coffee cake						■

FOOD	ALKALINE-FORMING			ACID-FORMING		
	High	Medium	Low	Low	Medium	High
Cupcakes, all flavors						■
Devil's food cake, chocolate frosting						■
Donuts, all flavors						■
Yellow cake, chocolate frosting						■
Camembert cheese						■
Canola oil				■		
Cantaloupe (muskmelon)	■					
Carbonated soft drinks, most types (See inset on page 142.)						■
Cardamom seeds		■				
Carrot cake, cream cheese frosting						■
Carrot juice				■		
Carrots (commercial) *				■		
Carrots (organic) *			■			
Cashew butter		■				
Cashews				■		
Catfish					■	
Catsup (ketchup)					■	

*Note that while mineral-rich organic carrots are alkaline-forming, most commercially farmed carrots are lower in minerals and higher in sugar, and therefore tend to be slightly acid-forming.

FOOD	ALKALINE-FORMING			ACID-FORMING		
	High	Medium	Low	Low	Medium	High
Cauliflower		■				
Cayenne pepper			■			
Celery	■					
Celery seeds			■			
CEREALS. *See also* **Grains.**						
Bran cereal					■	
Bran flakes and raisins (sweetened)				■		
Bran flakes and raisins (unsweetened)				■		
Buckwheat, whole grain				■		
Corn flakes					■	
Corn flakes, sugared (frosted)					■	
Farina						■
Granola (sweetened)				■		
Granola (unsweetened)			■			
Grits, corn						■
Grits, soy						■
Kasha				■		
Oat bran					■	
Oatmeal (sweetened)				■		
Oatmeal (unsweetened)			■			

FOOD	ALKALINE-FORMING			ACID-FORMING		
	High	Medium	Low	Low	Medium	High
Rice, puffed brown				■		
Rice, puffed white					■	
Chamomile tea			■			
Chard, Swiss				■		
Cheddar cheese (aged)						■
Cheesecake						■
CHEESES						
American cheese						■
Camembert						■
Cheddar cheese (aged)					■	
Cottage cheese					■	
Cream cheese					■	
Curd cheese				■		
Gouda						■
Hard cheese, most types						■
Mozzarella						■
Soft cheese, full-fat, most types					■	
Swiss cheese (aged)						■

FOOD	ALKALINE-FORMING			ACID-FORMING		
	High	Medium	Low	Low	Medium	High
Cherimoya				■		
Cherries		■				
Chestnuts	■					
Chicken						
liver					■	
meat					■	
Chicken noodle soup						■
Chicken nuggets, fried						■
Chicken sandwich, broiled						■
Chicken sandwich, fried						■
Chickpeas (garbanzo beans)				■		
Chili with beef						■
Chinese parsley (cilantro, coriander leaf)		■				
CHIPS						
Corn, fried						■
Potato, baked			■			
Potato, fried						■
Tortilla, fried						■

Chocolate *See also* Cocoa powder.

FOOD	ALKALINE-FORMING			ACID-FORMING		
	High	Medium	Low	Low	Medium	High
baking						■
dark						■
milk						■
Chocolate milk, whole cow's milk					■	
Cider, apple		■				
Cilantro (Chinese parsley, coriander leaf)		■				
Cinnamon		■				
CITRUS FRUITS						
Grapefruit		■				
Lemons		■				
Limes	■					
Mandarin oranges	■					
Oranges		■				
Tangelos		■				
Tangerines	■					
Clams				■		
Clarified butter (ghee)			■			
Cocoa powder						■
Coconut oil			■			

FOOD	ALKALINE-FORMING			ACID-FORMING		
	High	Medium	Low	Low	Medium	High
Coconuts			■			
Cod liver oil			■			
Coffee (See inset on page 100.)						
decaffeinated (water decaffeinated)					■	
espresso						■
regular					■	
Coffee cake						■
Cola drink (See page 142.)						■
Cold cuts *See* Luncheon Meat; Meat.						
Coleslaw				■		
Collard greens	■					
CONDIMENTS. *See also* Salad Dressings.						
Horseradish	■					
Ketchup (catsup)					■	
Mayonnaise				■		
Miso (soybean paste)	■					
Mustard, prepared					■	
Pickle relish						
Soy sauce (tamari)		■				

Coffee

Coffee is acidifying, a fact that many people experience in the form of an acidic stomach soon after they drink it. As a pick-me-up first thing in the morning and later in the day, however, coffee is one of the most commonly consumed beverages in the United States, as well as many other countries.

The primary reason for coffee's acidifying effect appears to be its acidifying organic acids and its caffeine. Many health experts, including Dr. Robert Anderson, MD, founding president of the American Board of Holistic Medicine, believe that more than 50 percent of American adults are addicted to caffeine, which is also found in chocolate, cocoa, colas, and many commercial teas. However, even decaffeinated coffee is acidifying. Further, consuming coffee causes a loss of minerals in the urine and contributes to a lack of hydration.

If you are a coffee drinker, be sure to increase the amount of alkalizing foods you eat each day, and to drink plenty of mineral water or pure filtered water. Another good option is water flavored with the juice of a lemon or lime, which is both tasty and highly alkalizing. Fortunately, as you shift towards eating more alkalizing foods, you may notice that your need for coffee decreases as your energy levels naturally start to rise.

	ALKALINE-FORMING			ACID-FORMING		
FOOD	High	Medium	Low	Low	Medium	High
COOKIES. *See also* Cakes; Desserts.						
Brownies						■
Chocolate chip, homemade						■
Sugar, homemade						■
Vanilla, homemade						■
Coriander leaf (Chinese parsley, cilantro)		■				
Coriander seeds			■			
Corn					■	
Corn chips, fried					■	■
Corn flakes					■	
Corn flakes, sugared (frosted)						■
Corn grits					■	
Corn syrup					■	■
Corn tortillas					■	
Cornmeal					■	
Cottage cheese					■	
Cottonseed meal						■
Cottonseed oil						■

	ALKALINE-FORMING			ACID-FORMING		
FOOD	High	Medium	Low	Low	Medium	High
Couscous, white flour *See also* Pasta.						■
Cow's milk *See* Milk.						
Crabs					■	
CRACKERS						
Matzoh						
white flour						■
whole wheat flour					■	
Rye crackers (100%)					■	
Saltine crackers						■
Whole wheat crackers					■	
Cranberries					■	
Cranberry sauce (sweetened)						■
Cream				■		
Cream, sour				■		
Cream cheese					■	
Croissants						■
Croutons (white flour)						■
Cucumbers *See also* Pickles.			■			
Cumin seeds		■				

FOOD	ALKALINE-FORMING			ACID-FORMING		
	High	Medium	Low	Low	Medium	High
Cupcakes, all flavors *See also* Cakes.						■
Curd cheese				■		
Currants		■				
Curry powder				■		
Daikon radish	■					
Dandelion greens		■				
Dates				■		
DESSERTS						
Angel food cake						■
Apple crisp (with oatmeal and Sucanat)			■			
Baked apples (sweetened)		■				
Baked apples (unsweetened)		■				
Brownies						■
Carrot cake, cream cheese frosting						■
Cheesecake						■
Coffee cake						■
Cookies						
chocolate chip, homemade						■
sugar, homemade						■
vanilla, homemade						■

FOOD	ALKALINE-FORMING			ACID-FORMING		
	High	Medium	Low	Low	Medium	High
Cupcakes, all flavors						■
Devil's food cake, chocolate frosting						■
Donuts, all flavors						■
Frozen tofu dessert						■
Ice cream, all flavors						■
Pies, fruit						
commercial, most flavors (highly sweetened)						■
homemade, most flavors (lightly sweetened)					■	
Puddings, most brands and flavors						■
Yellow cake, chocolate frosting						■
Yogurt, frozen, most brands						■
Yogurt, unfrozen. *See* Yogurt.						
Dill pickles, with apple cider vinegar		■				
Dill seeds			■			
Dill weed		■				
Donuts, all flavors						■
Dressings, salad *See* Salad Dressings.						

FOOD	ALKALINE-FORMING			ACID-FORMING		
	High	Medium	Low	Low	Medium	High
DRIED FRUITS						
Apricots				■		
Cranberries					■	
Dates				■		
Figs				■		
Prunes				■		
Raisins		■				
Duck					■	
Dulse seaweed *See also* Seaweed.	■					
Egg noodles, white flour *See also* Pasta.						■
Eggplant		■				
Eggs						
whites only				■		
whole					■	
Endive	■					
Evian water *See also* Mineral water, bottled.			■			
Farina cereal						■
FATS AND OILS						
Avocado oil			■			

FOOD	ALKALINE-FORMING High	Medium	Low	ACID-FORMING Low	Medium	High
Butter				■		
Canola oil				■		
Clarified butter (ghee)			■			
Coconut oil			■			
Cod liver oil			■			
Cottonseed oil			■			■
Flaxseed oil			■			
Lard					■	
Macadamia oil			■			
Margarine, most brands			■			
Olive oil			■			
Peanut oil			■		■	
Primrose oil			■			
Safflower oil				■		
Sesame oil				■		
Soybean oil				■	■	
Sunflower oil				■		
Vegetable oil, most types				■		
Fava beans				■		

FOOD	ALKALINE-FORMING			ACID-FORMING		
	High	Medium	Low	Low	Medium	High
Fennel seeds		■				
Figs				■		
Fiji water *See also* Mineral water, bottled.			■			
Filberts (hazelnuts) *See also* Hazelnut butter.						■
FISH AND SEAFOOD						
Bass					■	
Catfish					■	
Clams				■		
Crabs					■	
Flounder					■	
Grouper					■	
Haddock					■	
Halibut					■	
Herring, pickled					■	
Lobster					■	■
Mackerel					■	
Mussels					■	■
Orange roughy					■	
Oysters					■	
Perch					■	

FOOD	ALKALINE-FORMING			ACID-FORMING		
	High	Medium	Low	Low	Medium	High
Perch, white					■	
Pike					■	
Pollack (pollock)					■	
Salmon					■	
Scallops					■	
Scrod					■	
Sea bass					■	
Shrimp						■
Snapper					■	
Swordfish						■
Tuna					■	
Turbot					■	
Whitefish					■	
Whiting					■	
Yellowtail					■	
Fish fillet sandwich, fried						■
Flaxseed			■			
Flaxseed oil			■			
Flounder					■	

FOOD	ALKALINE-FORMING			ACID-FORMING		
	High	Medium	Low	Low	Medium	High
FLOUR						
Amaranth flour				■		
Barley flour					■	
Buckwheat flour				■		
Millet flour				■		
Oat flour			■			
Rice flour, brown				■		
Rice flour, white						■
Rye flour					■	
Soy flour						■
Triticale flour				■		
Wheat flour, white						■
Whole wheat flour					■	
Frankfurters						
beef						■
beef, on a bun						■
pork					■	
pork, on a bun						■
turkey				■		

	ALKALINE-FORMING			ACID-FORMING		
FOOD	High	Medium	Low	Low	Medium	High
vegetarian (soy and bean)						■
French dressing *See also* Salad Dressings.				■		
French fried onion rings						■
French fried potatoes						■
Fried foods in general						■
FRUIT JUICES						
Apple cider		■				
Apple juice (sweetened)			■	■		
Apple juice (unsweetened)			■			
Berry juice blend			■			
Grape juice			■			
Grapefruit juice		■				
Lemon juice	■					
Lime juice	■					
Orange juice			■			
Pear juice			■			
Pineapple juice		■				
Tomato juice or juice blend				■		

FOOD	ALKALINE-FORMING			ACID-FORMING		
	High	Medium	Low	Low	Medium	High
Fruit preserves, jams, and jellies, all flavors (sweetened with sugar or corn syrup)						■
FRUITS						
Apples						
baked (sweetened)		■				
baked (unsweetened)			■			
raw		■				
Apricots		■				
Avocados		■				
Bananas		■				
Blackberries	■					
Blueberries	■					
Boysenberries	■					
Cantaloupe (muskmelon)	■					
Cherimoya				■		
Cherries		■				
Coconuts			■			
Currants		■				
Dates				■		

FOOD	ALKALINE-FORMING			ACID-FORMING		
	High	Medium	Low	Low	Medium	High
Figs				■		
Grapefruits		■				
Grapes		■				
Guava				■		
Honeydew melon	■					
Kiwi fruit	■					
Lemons		■				
Limes	■					
Mandarin oranges	■					
Mangos	■					
Olives						
green		■				
ripe					■	
Oranges		■				
Papayas	■					
Peaches		■				
Pears		■				
Persimmon	■					
Pineapples	■					
Plums				■		

FOOD	ALKALINE-FORMING			ACID-FORMING		
	High	Medium	Low	Low	Medium	High
Pomegranates					■	
Prunes				■		
Raisins		■				
Raspberries	■					
Strawberries	■					
Tangelos		■				
Tangerines	■					
Tomatoes				■		
Watermelons	■					
Garbanzo beans (chickpeas)				■		
Garlic		■				
Gelatin				■		
Ghee (clarified butter)			■			
Gin						■
Ginger root	■					
Ginger tea	■					
Goat					■	
Goat's milk				■		
Gouda cheese						■

FOOD	ALKALINE-FORMING			ACID-FORMING		
	High	Medium	Low	Low	Medium	High
GRAINS. *See also* **Cereals; Flour.**						
Barley, whole grain					■	
Bulgur wheat (hard red winter)					■	
Corn					■	
Cornmeal					■	
Cottonseed meal						■
Grits, corn					■	
Kasha (buckwheat groats)				■		
Malt						■
Millet				■		
Oat bran					■	
Quinoa			■			
Rice						
brown rice				■		
japonica rice			■			
white rice					■	
wild rice			■			
Rye					■	
Teff				■		
Triticale, whole grain				■		

FOOD	ALKALINE-FORMING			ACID-FORMING		
	High	Medium	Low	Low	Medium	High
Wheat, unrefined				■		
Granola (sweetened)				■		
Granola (unsweetened)			■			
Granulated sugar (white) See also Sugar.						■
Grapes		■				
Grape juice		■	■			
Grapefruit		■				
Grapefruit juice		■				
Great Northern beans				■		
Green beans See String, green, snap, wax, and yellow beans.						
Green bell peppers		■				
Green onions (scallions)		■				
Green tea, most types			■			
Greens, leafy See Leafy Greens.						
Grits						
corn					■	
soy						■
Grouper					■	
Guava				■		

FOOD	ALKALINE-FORMING			ACID-FORMING		
	High	Medium	Low	Low	Medium	High
Haddock					▓	
Halibut					▓	
Ham						
pork					▓	
turkey				▓		
Hamburgers						
beef						▓
beef, on a bun						▓
beef with cheese, on a bun						▓
turkey					▓	
vegetarian, few beans					▓	
vegetarian, mostly beans				▓		
vegetarian, mostly whole grains				▓		
vegetarian, mostly soy (tofu)						▓
Hard cheeses, most types *See also* Cheeses.						
Hash brown potatoes			▓			
Hazelnut butter						▓
Hazelnuts (filberts)						▓
Herbal teas, most types			▓			

FOOD	ALKALINE-FORMING			ACID-FORMING		
	High	Medium	Low	Low	Medium	High
HERBS AND SPICES (FRESH AND DRIED)						
Basil		■				
Bay leaf			■			
Cardamon seeds		■				
Celery seeds			■			
Cilantro		■				
Cinnamon		■				
Coriander seeds			■			
Cumin seeds			■			
Curry powder				■		
Dill seeds			■			
Dill weed		■				
Fennel seeds		■				
Ginger root	■					
Mace			■			
Marjoram		■				
Oregano		■				
Paprika	■					
Parsley	■					
Pepper						

FOOD	ALKALINE-FORMING			ACID-FORMING		
	High	Medium	Low	Low	Medium	High
black		■				
cayenne			■			
Salt						
iodized table						■
sea	■					
Tarragon		■				
Thyme		■				
Watercress		■				
Herring, pickled					■	
Hijiki seaweed *See also* Seaweed.	■					
Home fries (potatoes), homemade			■			
Honey				■		
Honeydew melon	■					
Hops						■
Horseradish	■					
Hot dogs						
beef						■
beef, on a bun						■
pork					■	

FOOD	ALKALINE-FORMING			ACID-FORMING		
	High	Medium	Low	Low	Medium	High
pork, on a bun						■
turkey					■	
vegetarian (soy and bean)						■
Hubbard squash		■				
Hummus				■		
Ice cream, all flavors						■
Iodized table salt *See also* Salt.						■
Irish moss seaweed *See also* Seaweed.			■			
Italian dressing, with olive oil and apple cider vinegar *See also* Salad Dressings.			■			
Jams, jellies, and preserves, all flavors (sweetened with sugar or corn syrup)						■
Japonica rice			■			
Jerusalem artichoke		■				
Jicama			■			
Juices *See* Fruit Juices; Vegetable Juices.						
Kale	■					
Kasha (buckwheat groats)				■		
Kefir (fermented cow's milk)				■		
Kelp *See also* Seaweed.	■					

FOOD	ALKALINE-FORMING			ACID-FORMING		
	High	Medium	Low	Low	Medium	High
Ketchup (catsup)					■	
Kidney beans				■		
Kielbasa sausage					■	
Kiwi fruit	■					
Knockwurst sausage, link					■	
Kohlrabi	■					
Kombu seaweed *See also* Seaweed.	■					
Kraut (sauerkraut)		■				
Lamb					■	
Lard					■	
Lasagna						■
LEAFY GREENS						
Chard Swiss				■		
Collard greens	■					
Dandelion greens		■				
Kale	■					
Lettuce						
iceberg		■				
red leaf		■				
romaine		■				

FOOD	ALKALINE-FORMING			ACID-FORMING		
	High	Medium	Low	Low	Medium	High
Mustard greens	■					
Salad greens, mixed		■				
Spinach				■		
Turnip greens		■				
Legumes *See* Beans and Legumes.						
Lemon juice	■					
Lemons		■				
Lentils		■				
Lettuce						
iceberg		■				
red leaf		■				
romaine		■				
Lima beans (butter beans)				■		
Lime juice	■					
Limes	■					
Linguine, white flour *See also* Pasta.						■
Liver						
beef					■	
chicken					■	

FOOD	ALKALINE-FORMING			ACID-FORMING		
	High	Medium	Low	Low	Medium	High
Liverwurst					■	
Lotus root	■					
Lobster						■
LUNCHEON MEAT						
Beef sausage						■
Bologna, beef						■
Bologna, bratwurst, link					■	
Bologna, turkey					■	
Corned beef						■
Frankfurters						
beef						■
pork					■	
turkey					■	
vegetarian (soy and bean)						■
Ham, pork					■	
Ham, turkey					■	
Kielbasa sausage					■	
Knockwurst sausage, link					■	
Liverwurst					■	
Pastrami					■	

FOOD	ALKALINE-FORMING			ACID-FORMING		
	High	Medium	Low	Low	Medium	High
Pepperoni					■	
Pork sausage						■
Salami, pork or beef						■
Turkey breast					■	
Macadamia nuts			■			
Macadamia oil			■			
Macaroni, white flour *See also* Pasta.						■
Macaroni and Cheese						■
Mace			■			
Mackerel					■	
Malt						■
Malt liquor						
dark					■	
pale						■
Mandarin oranges	■					
Mangos	■					
Maple syrup				■		
Marjoram		■				

FOOD	ALKALINE-FORMING			ACID-FORMING		
	High	Medium	Low	Low	Medium	High
Matzoh						
white flour						■
whole wheat flour					■	
Mayonnaise				■		
MEAT. *See also* Fish; Luncheon Meat; Poultry.						
Beef						
bologna						■
frankfurters						■
hamburgers						■
liver					■	
meat (steak, roasts, etc.)						■
sausage						■
Buffalo (bison)					■	
Goat					■	
Lamb					■	
Pork						
bacon, fried						■
frankfurters					■	
ham					■	
lard					■	

FOOD	ALKALINE-FORMING			ACID-FORMING		
	High	Medium	Low	Low	Medium	High
meat (chops, roasts, etc.)					■	
sausage					■	
Rabbit					■	
Veal						■
Venison					■	

Melons

FOOD	ALKALINE-FORMING			ACID-FORMING		
cantaloupe	■					
honeydew	■					
watermelon	■					

Milk *See also* Almond milk; Rice milk; Soy milk.

FOOD	ALKALINE-FORMING			ACID-FORMING		
cow's milk, skim (nonfat)					■	
cow's milk, 1% fat					■	
cow's milk, 2% fat					■	
cow's milk, whole					■	
cow's milk, chocolate-flavored, whole				■	■	
goat's milk				■		
kefir (fermented cow's milk)				■		

Milk shakes, commercial

FOOD	ALKALINE-FORMING			ACID-FORMING		
chocolate						■

FOOD	ALKALINE-FORMING			ACID-FORMING		
	High	Medium	Low	Low	Medium	High
vanilla	•					■

Milk substitute *See* Almond milk; Rice milk; Soy milk.

Millet				■		
Millet flour				■		

Mineral water, bottled *See also* Tap water.

Apollinaris	■					
Evian			■			
Fiji	■					
San Pellegrino	■					
Sanfaustino	■					
Volvic			■			
Miso	■					
Molasses		■				
Monosodium glutamate (MSG)				■		
Mozzarella cheese						■
MSG (monosodium glutamate)				■		
Mung beans				■		
Mushrooms			■			
Muskmelon (cantaloupe)	■					
Mussels						■

FOOD	ALKALINE-FORMING			ACID-FORMING		
	High	Medium	Low	Low	Medium	High
Mustard, prepared					■	
Mustard greens	■					
Navy beans				■		
Noodles, egg *See also* Pasta.						■
Nori seaweed *See also* Seaweed.	■					
NUT BUTTERS						
Almond butter			■			
Cashew butter		■				
Hazelnut butter						■
Peanut butter					■	
Pistachio butter					■	
Nut milk, almond (sweetened)			■	■		
Nut milk, almond (unsweetened)				■		
NUTS AND SEEDS						
Almonds			■			
Amaranth seeds. *See also* Flour.				■		
Cashews		■				
Celery seeds			■			

FOOD	ALKALINE-FORMING			ACID-FORMING		
	High	Medium	Low	Low	Medium	High
Chestnuts	■					
Coriander seeds			■			
Cumin seeds		■				
Flaxseed			■			
Hazelnuts (filberts)						■
Macadamia nuts			■			
Peanuts					■	
Pecans					■	
Pine nuts				■		
Pistachio nuts					■	
Pumpkin seeds	■					
Quinoa seeds			■			
Sesame seeds			■			
Soy nuts						■
Sunflower seeds			■			
Walnuts						■
Oat bran					■	
Oat flour			■			
Oats and oatmeal (sweetened)				■		

FOOD	ALKALINE-FORMING			ACID-FORMING		
	High	Medium	Low	Low	Medium	High
Oats and oatmeal (unsweetened)			■			
Oils *See* Fats and Oils.						
Okra		■				
Olive oil			■			
Olives						
green		■				
ripe					■	
Onions	■					
Onions, green (scallions)		■				
Orange juice			■			
Orange roughy					■	
Oranges		■				
Oranges, mandarin	■					
Oregano		■				
Oysters					■	
Pancakes, white flour						■
Papayas	■					
Paprika	■					
Parsley	■					
Parsnips	■					

FOOD	ALKALINE-FORMING			ACID-FORMING		
	High	Medium	Low	Low	Medium	High
PASTA						
Couscous, white flour						■
Egg noodles, white flour						■
Linguine, white flour						■
Macaroni, white flour						■
Spaghetti						
rye flour					■	
white flour						■
whole wheat flour					■	
Pasta sauce (tomato based)						
with meat					■	
without meat				■		
Pastrami						
PASTRY. *See also* **Desserts.**						
Danish, cheese						■
Puff pastry						■
Peas						
fresh green				■		

FOOD	ALKALINE-FORMING			ACID-FORMING		
	High	Medium	Low	Low	Medium	High
split peas, green and yellow				■		
Peas, snow			■			
Peaches		■				
Peanut butter					■	
Peanut oil					■	
Peanuts					■	
Pear juice			■			
Pears		■				
Pecans					■	
Pellegrino water *See also* Mineral water, bottled.	■					
Pepper (spice)						
black		■				
cayenne pepper			■			
Pepperoni					■	
Peppers, bell (sweet)						
green		■				
red		■				
yellow		■				
Peppers, hot		■				
Perch					■	

FOOD	ALKALINE-FORMING			ACID-FORMING		
	High	Medium	Low	Low	Medium	High
Perch, white					■	
Persimmon	■					
Phosphoric acid (commercial flavoring)						■
Pickles						
dill, with apple cider vinegar		■				
sweet, with white vinegar and sugar					■	
PIES, FRUIT						
Commercial, most flavors (highly sweetened)						■
Homemade, most flavors (lightly sweetened)					■	
Pike					■	
Pine nuts				■		
Pineapple juice		■				
Pineapples	■					
Pinto beans				■		
Pistachio butter					■	
Pistachio nuts					■	
Pita bread, white						■
Pita bread, whole wheat					■	

FOOD	ALKALINE-FORMING			ACID-FORMING		
	High	Medium	Low	Low	Medium	High
Pizza						
cheese						■
marinara (no cheese)						■
pepperoni						■
Plums				■		
Pollack (pollock)					■	
Pomegranates					■	
Popcorn					■	
Popcorn cakes *See also* Rice cakes.					■	
Pork *See also* Luncheon meats.						
bacon						■
frankfurters					■	
ham					■	
lard					■	
meat (chops, roasts, etc.)					■	
sausage					■	
Pork and beans, baked *See also* Baked beans.					■	
Potato chips						
baked			■			
fried						■

FOOD	ALKALINE-FORMING			ACID-FORMING		
	High	Medium	Low	Low	Medium	High
Potatoes						
baked, skin on		■				
French fried, commercial						■
home fries, homemade			■			
mashed, with milk and butter		■				
Potatoes, sweet	■					
POULTRY						
Chicken						
liver					■	
meat					■	
Duck					■	
Turkey					■	
bologna					■	
frankfurters					■	
ham					■	
meat					■	
Preservatives						
Benzoate					■	

FOOD	ALKALINE-FORMING			ACID-FORMING		
	High	Medium	Low	Low	Medium	High
Preserves, jams, and jellies, all flavors (sweetened with sugar or corn sweetener)						■
Pretzels, white flour						■
Primrose oil			■			
Prunes				■		
Puddings, most brands and flavors						■
Pumpernickel bread					■	
Pumpkin seeds	■					
Quiche, all types						■
Quinoa			■			
Rabbit					■	
Radishes	■					
Radishes, daikon	■					
Raisins		■				
Raspberries	■					
Red bell peppers		■				
Red wine					■	
Red wine vinegar						■
Rhubarb				■		

FOOD	ALKALINE-FORMING			ACID-FORMING		
	High	Medium	Low	Low	Medium	High
Rice						
brown rice				■		
japonica rice			■			
white rice					■	
wild rice			■			
Rice cakes *See also* Popcorn cakes.						
brown rice, multigrain				■		
brown rice, plain					■	
white rice					■	
Rice cereal, puffed brown				■		
Rice cereal, puffed white					■	
Rice flour						
brown				■		
white						■
Rice milk					■	
Rice syrup			■			
Rice vinegar				■		
Roast beef sandwich						■
Root beer				■		
Russian dressing *See also* Salad Dressings.				■		

FOOD	ALKALINE-FORMING			ACID-FORMING		
	High	Medium	Low	Low	Medium	High
Rutabagas	■					
Rye					■	
Rye bread (100%)					■	
Rye crackers (100%)					■	
Rye flour					■	
Saccharin					■	
Safflower oil				■		
SALAD DRESSINGS. *See also* Condiments; Fats and Oils; Vinegars.						
Caesar						■
French				■		
Italian, with olive oil and apple cider vinegar			■			
Russian				■		
Thousand Island				■		
Salad greens, mixed		■				
Salami, pork or beef						■
Salmon					■	
Salt						
iodized table salt						■
sea salt	■					

FOOD	ALKALINE-FORMING			ACID-FORMING		
	High	Medium	Low	Low	Medium	High
Saltine crackers						■
Sanfaustino water *See also* Mineral water, bottled.	■					
SAUCES						
Catsup (ketchup)					■	
Cranberry sauce (sweetened)						■
Soy sauce (tamari)		■				
Spaghetti sauce (tomato based)						
with meat					■	
without meat				■		
Tomato sauce						
with meat					■	
without meat						
Sauerkraut		■				
Sausages *See also* Luncheon Meat.						
beef						■
kielbasa					■	
knockwurst, link					■	
pork					■	
Scallions (green onions)		■				

FOOD	ALKALINE-FORMING			ACID-FORMING		
	High	Medium	Low	Low	Medium	High
Scallops					■	
Scotch						■
Scrod					■	
Sea bass					■	
Sea salt	■					
Seaweed						
agar		■				
dulse	■					
hijiki	■					
Irish moss			■			
kelp	■					
kombu	■					
nori		■				
spirulina			■			
wakame	■					
SEEDS						
Amaranth seeds				■		
Celery seeds			■			
Coriander seeds			■			
Cumin seeds		■				

FOOD	ALKALINE-FORMING			ACID-FORMING		
	High	Medium	Low	Low	Medium	High
Flaxseed			■			
Pumpkin seeds	■					
Quinoa seeds			■			
Sesame seeds			■			
Sunflower seeds			■			
Sesame butter (tahini sauce)			■			
Sesame oil				■		
Sesame seeds			■			
SHELLFISH *See also* **Fish and Seafood.**						
Clams				■		
Crabs					■	
Lobster						■
Mussels						■
Oysters					■	
Scallops					■	
Shrimp						■
Shrimp						■
Skim milk *See also* Milk.				■		

FOOD	ALKALINE-FORMING			ACID-FORMING		
	High	Medium	Low	Low	Medium	High
SNACK FOODS *See also* Crackers; Desserts; Nuts and Seeds.						
Corn chips, fried						■
Popcorn					■	
Popcorn cakes					■	
Potato chips						
baked			■			
fried						■
Pretzels, white flour						■
Rice cakes						
brown rice, multigrain				■		
brown rice, plain				■		
white rice					■	
Soy nuts						■
Tortilla chips, fried						■
Snap beans *See* String, green, snap, wax, and yellow beans.						
Snapper					■	
Snow peas			■			
Soft drinks (carbonated), most types (See inset on page 142.)						■

Carbonated Soft Drinks

Carbonated soft drinks are among the most acidifying substances found in the supermarket. Researcher Sang Whang, author of the book *Reverse Aging,* has found that to neutralize the acidifying effects of one glass of soda, the average person needs to drink *thirty-two glasses of highly alkaline water!* And unfortunately, the consumption of soft drinks has increased dramatically over the past several years, with Americans now consuming about two cans a day per person.

What makes carbonated soft drinks so acidifying? A number of ingredients are to blame. Nearly all soft drinks, for instance, contain phosphoric acid and caffeine, both of which have an acidifying effect on the body. Regular (nondiet) sodas also feature an abundance of corn syrup and/or sugar, which, too, are highly acid-forming. (See pages 101 and 146 of the table.) And if you think that diet sodas are any better, think again, because artificial sweeteners such as aspartame and saccharin also tilt the body's pH into the acid range. (See page 82.)

Clearly, if your goal is to create a healthy alkaline environment in your body, you should avoid drinking soda altogether. If your craving for soft drinks persists, consider soda substitutes such as club soda or unflavored seltzer water, or "health food" sodas made without phosphoric acid and sweeteners. Keep in mind, though, that even these products should be consumed only sparingly.

	ALKALINE-FORMING			ACID-FORMING		
FOOD	High	Medium	Low	Low	Medium	High
SOUPS						
Black bean soup				■		
Borscht		■				
Chicken noodle soup						■
Split pea soup				■		
Tomato soup				■		
Vegetable soup			■			
Sour cream				■		
Soy flour						■
Soy grits						■
Soy milk, most brands						■
Soy nuts						■
Soy protein						
concentrate						■
isolate						■
Soy sauce (tamari)		■				
Soybean curd (tofu), all types						■
Soybean oil					■	
Soybean paste (miso)	■					

	ALKALINE-FORMING			ACID-FORMING		
FOOD	High	Medium	Low	Low	Medium	High
Soybeans						■
Spaghetti						
rye flour					■	
white flour						■
whole wheat flour					■	
Spaghetti sauce (tomato based)						
with meat					■	
without meat				■		
Spices *See* Herbs and Spices.						
Spinach				■		
Spirulina seaweed *See also* Seaweed.			■			
Split pea soup				■		
Split peas, green and yellow				■		
SPREADS *See also* Cheeses; Condiments.						
Almond butter			■			
Apple butter		■				
Butter				■		
Cashew butter		■				
Cream cheese					■	
Hazelnut butter						■

FOOD	ALKALINE-FORMING			ACID-FORMING		
	High	Medium	Low	Low	Medium	High
Hummus				■		
Jams, jellies, and preserves, all flavors (sweetened with sugar or corn syrup)						■
Peanut butter					■	
Pistachio butter					■	
Spring onions (scallions)		■				
Spring water *See* Mineral water, bottled.						
Sprouts, most types			■			
bean sprouts		■				
Squash						
Hubbard squash		■				
summer squash		■				
winter squash	■					
zucchini		■				
Steak, beef						■
Stevia				■		
Strawberries	■					
String, green, snap, wax, and yellow beans, *with* formed beans				■		

FOOD	ALKALINE-FORMING			ACID-FORMING		
	High	Medium	Low	Low	Medium	High
String, green, snap, wax, and yellow beans, *without* formed beans		■				
Sucanat sweetener, organic			■			
Sugar						
brown sugar						■
Sucanat, organic			■			
white sugar (granulated)						■
Sugared (frosted) corn flakes					■	
Summer squash		■				
Sunflower oil				■		
Sunflower seeds			■			
Sweet pickles, with white vinegar and sugar					■	
Sweet potatoes	■					
SWEETENERS						
Artificial						
Aspartame					■	
Saccharin					■	
Corn syrup						■
Honey				■		
Maple syrup				■		

FOOD	ALKALINE-FORMING			ACID-FORMING		
	High	Medium	Low	Low	Medium	High
Molasses		■				
Rice syrup			■			
Stevia				■		
Sugar						
brown sugar						■
Sucanat, organic			■			
white sugar (granulated)						■
Swiss chard				■		
Swiss cheese (aged)						■
Swordfish						■
SYRUPS *See also* Sweeteners.						
Corn syrup						■
Maple syrup				■		
Rice syrup			■			
Tacos						
with beef						■
with chicken						
Tahini sauce (sesame butter)			■			

FOOD	ALKALINE-FORMING			ACID-FORMING		
	High	Medium	Low	Low	Medium	High
Tamari soy sauce		■				
Tangelos		■				
Tangerines	■					
Tap water *See also* Mineral water, bottled.						
chlorinated, in general				■		
nonchlorinated, in general*				■		
Taro root	■					
Tarragon		■				
Tea						
black tea, most types				■		
green tea, most types			■			
herbal tea, most types			■			
Teff				■		
Tempeh					■	
Thousand Island dressing *See also* Salad Dressings.				■		
Thyme		■				
Tofu, all types						■
Tofu frozen desserts, all types						■
Tomato juice or juice blend				■		

* Be aware that the value provided for nonchlorinated tap water is only an average, and that tap water can vary in its impact from region to region. See the inset on page 156 for more information.

FOOD	ALKALINE-FORMING			ACID-FORMING		
	High	Medium	Low	Low	Medium	High
Tomato paste (canned)				■		
Tomato sauce						
with meat					■	
without meat				■		
Tomato soup				■		
Tomatoes				■		
Tortilla chips, fried						■
Tortillas						
corn					■	
white flour						■
Triticale, whole grain				■		
Triticale flour				■		
Tuna, fresh or canned					■	
Turbot					■	
Turkey						
bologna					■	
ham					■	
meat					■	
Turnip greens		■				
Turnips		■				

FOOD	ALKALINE-FORMING			ACID-FORMING		
	High	Medium	Low	Low	Medium	High
Umeboshi vinegar	■					
Vanilla extract				■		
Veal						■
VEGETABLE JUICES						
Carrot juice				■		
Tomato juice or juice blend				■		
Vegetable juice cocktail (commercial), tomato based				■		
Vegetable juice cocktail (homemade), green vegetables with apple, no tomato	■					
Vegetable oil, most types *See also* Fats and Oils.				■		
Vegetable soup			■			
VEGETABLES						
Artichokes		■				
Artichokes, Jerusalem		■				
Asparagus	■	■				
Beets		■				
Bell peppers						
green		■				
red		■				

FOOD	ALKALINE-FORMING			ACID-FORMING		
	High	Medium	Low	Low	Medium	High
yellow		■				
Broccoli		■				
Brussels sprouts			■			
Burdock root	■					
Cabbage						
Chinese		■				
red		■				
white		■				
Carrots (commercial)*				■		
Carrots (organic)*			■			
Cauliflower		■				
Celery	■					
Chard, Swiss				■		
Collards	■					
Corn					■	
Cucumbers. *See also* Pickles.			■			
Dandelion greens		■				
Eggplant			■			
Endive	■					
Garlic		■				

*Note that while mineral-rich organic carrots are alkaline-forming, most commercially farmed carrots are lower in minerals and higher in sugar, and therefore tend to be slightly acid-forming.

FOOD	ALKALINE-FORMING			ACID-FORMING		
	High	Medium	Low	Low	Medium	High
Green onions (scallions)		■				
Jicama		■				
Kale	■					
Kohlrabi	■					
Lettuce						
iceberg		■				
red leaf		■				
romaine		■				
Lotus root	■					
Mushrooms			■			
Mustard greens	■					
Okra		■				
Onions	■					
Parsnips	■					
Peas						
fresh green				■		
split peas, green and yellow				■		
Potatoes		■				
Radishes	■					
Radishes, daikon	■					

FOOD	ALKALINE-FORMING			ACID-FORMING		
	High	Medium	Low	Low	Medium	High
Rhubarb				■		
Rutabagas	■					
Salad greens, mixed		■				
Snow peas			■			
Spinach				■		
Squash						
Hubbard squash		■				
summer squash		■				
winter squash	■					
zucchini		■				
String, green, snap, wax, and yellow beans, *with* formed beans				■		
String, green, snap, wax, and yellow beans, *without* formed beans		■				
Sweet potatoes	■					
Taro root	■					
Tomatoes				■		
Turnip greens		■				
Turnips		■				
Watercress		■				
Yams	■					

FOOD	ALKALINE-FORMING			ACID-FORMING		
	High	Medium	Low	Low	Medium	High
Zucchini		■				
Vegetarian burgers *See* Hamburgers.						
Venison					■	
Vinegars						
apple cider vinegar		■				
balsamic vinegar				■		
red wine vinegar						■
rice vinegar				■		
umeboshi vinegar	■					
white vinegar						■
Vodka						■
Volvic water *See also* Mineral water, bottled.			■			
Waffles, white flour						■
Wakame seaweed *See also* Seaweed.	■					
Walnuts						■
WATER (See inset on page 156.)						
Bottled mineral						
Apollinaris		■				
Evian			■			

	ALKALINE-FORMING			ACID-FORMING		
FOOD	High	Medium	Low	Low	Medium	High
Fiji			■			
San Pellegrino	■					
Sanfaustino	■					
Volvic			■			
Tap						
chlorinated, in general				■		
nonchlorinated, in general*				■		
Watercress		■				
Watermelon	■					
Wax beans *See* String, green, snap, wax, and yellow beans.						
Wheat, unrefined				■		
Wheat (bran) flakes and raisins (sweetened)				■		
Wheat (bran) flakes and raisins (unsweetened)				■		
Wheat flour						
white						■
whole wheat					■	
Whey						
cow			■			

* Be aware that the value provided for nonchlorinated tap water is only an average, and that tap water can vary in its impact from region to region. See the inset on page 156 for more information.

The pH of Drinking Water

Pure water has a pH value of 7.0, making it neutral. This means that it produces neither acidifying nor alkalizing effects within the body when it is consumed. Why, then, is the water in the food table on pages 154 to 155 *not* neutral? Because most drinking water is not pure and therefore does not have a neutral pH.

Even though the pH of drinking water is usually not neutral, water is not a significant factor in terms of encouraging metabolic acidosis. This is true because the total concentration of acids in tap water is very small. The fact is that even though a small amount of acid placed in water can lower the water's pH reading a great deal, the overall metabolic impact of that small amount of acid is not consequential.

There are, however, factors other than the pH reading of water that *are* important in terms of the water's impact on acid-alkaline balance. Chief among these are the following:

■ **The Concentration of Minerals.** The concentration of minerals in water is an important factor in determining its effects on the body's pH levels. One of the most common means of determining this level of concentration is to measure the amount of "dissolved solids" in water. Water that is highly mineralized, such as European mineral water, contains 1,500 or more milligrams of dissolved solids per liter. By comparison, most tap water contains only 50 milligrams or so of dissolved solids. Typically, such dissolved solids include alkalizing minerals such as calcium and magnesium, as well as alkalizing bicarbonates. (In some cases, they can also include acidifying dissolved solids such as chloride, however.)

Alkalizing minerals and bicarbonate in water can have a significant impact on acid-base balance, as they are readily taken up into the body. As obtained from mineral water, bicarbonate and alkalizing forms of calcium and magnesium have been shown to reduce both urinary calcium loss and bone breakdown.

■ **Chloride Content.** The chloride content of water is another important factor in determining its impact on pH. It is important to note, for instance, that the amount of calcium and magnesium that water contains is not as important as whether these minerals occur in the form of calcium and magnesium *chloride*. Why? Because while nonchloride forms of calcium and magnesium increase alkalinity, chloride forms increase acidity. The healthiest types of water have the lowest levels of chloride.

■ **Bicarbonate Content.** Bicarbonate is an ion of carbonic acid in which one of the hydrogen atoms has been replaced by a metal such as sodium. Bicarbonate has an alkalizing effect, and the amount of bicarbonate present in the blood has been found to be an indicator of the body's reserves of alkalizing minerals. Those mineral waters that are high in alkalizing bicarbonates of calcium and magnesium have been shown to slow bone loss—often an effect of chronic acidosis—independent of the alkalizing impact of the calcium-containing foods. In addition, overall, the alkalizing minerals and bicarbonates contained in mineral water are much more easily assimilated by the body, compared with the minerals found in food. The mineral and bicarbonate levels of mineral waters can vary quite a bit, depending on the water's origin.

Each of the above three factors needs to be considered when determining the effects that drinking water will have on your body's metabolic acid-alkaline balance. If you rely on municipal tap water for your drinking needs, you can obtain information on the amount of dissolved solids, chloride, and bicarbonates contained in your water by contacting your local water board. Keep in mind that you don't want to know the water's pH, as this is a poor indication of its effect on the body. You want information on dissolved solids. If the water in your area is chlorinated, though, you can be sure that it is acid-forming.

If you drink bottled mineral water, simply contact the supplier, as most will be glad to tell you the mineral content of their product. It's worth the effort, because mineral water high in dissolved solids and bicarbonates and low in chloride is an effective means of correcting chronic low-grade metabolic acidosis and building mineral reserves.

FOOD	ALKALINE-FORMING			ACID-FORMING		
	High	Medium	Low	Low	Medium	High
goat			■			
White beans				■		
White bread						■
White perch					■	
White rice					■	
White rice cakes					■	
White rice flour						■
White sugar (granulated) *See also* Sugar.						■
White vinegar						■
White wine					■	
Whitefish					■	
Whiting					■	
Whole wheat bread					■	
Whole wheat crackers					■	
Wieners *See* Frankfurters.						
Wild rice			■			
Wine						
red					■	
white					■	
Winter squash	■					

FOOD	ALKALINE-FORMING			ACID-FORMING		
	High	Medium	Low	Low	Medium	High
Yams	■					
Yeast						■
Yellow beans *See* String, green, snap, wax, and yellow beans.						
Yellow bell peppers		■				
Yellow cake, chocolate frosting						■
Yellowtail					■	
Yogurt						
cow's milk (sweetened)				■		■
cow's milk (unsweetened)				■		
goat's milk (sweetened)				■		■
goat's milk (unsweetened)				■		
sheep's milk (sweetened)				■		■
sheep's milk (unsweetened)				■		
soy (sweetened)				■		■
soy (unsweetened)						■
Yogurt, frozen, most brands						■
Zucchini		■				

FAST FOOD TABLE

The following table is a quick guide to the acidifying and alkalizing effects of some of the most common and popular fast food items. As you can see, most fast foods, by their very nature, are highly acidifying for several reasons. First, fast foods are highly processed and, as a result, are low in alkalizing minerals. Further, they often contain various ingredients—food colorings and dyes, flavorings, preservatives, sweeteners, and unhealthy fats and oils—that have an acidifying effect on the body.

To ensure good health, you should avoid fast foods altogether. If, however, you find yourself on the go and unable to prepare or purchase a healthier meal, you can combine selected parts of the fast food menu to keep acidity in check. For example, a combination of broiled chicken without the bun, a salad, and a baked potato would be low acid-forming or even alkalizing, depending on the portion sizes. Also try to ensure that you have enough alkali reserves to deal with the acid load imposed by fast foods. The best way to do this is to make sure your everyday diet is high in fruits, vegetables, nuts, and seeds; to drink alkalizng mineral water; and to use alkalizing mineral supplements as necessary.

FAST FOOD TABLE

FOOD	ALKALINE-FORMING			ACID-FORMING		
	High	Medium	Low	Low	Medium	High
ENTRÉES						
Burrito						
with beef						■
with chicken						■
Chicken nuggets, fried						■
Chicken sandwich, broiled						■
Chicken sandwich, fried						■
Chili with beef						■
Fish fillet sandwich, fried						■
Frankfurter (beef) on a bun						■
Frankfurter (pork) on a bun						■
Hamburger, vegetarian. *See* Hamburgers on page 116.						
Hamburger (beef) on a bun						■
Hamburger (beef) with cheese on a bun						■
Pizza with sauce and cheese						■
Roast beef sandwich						■
Taco						
with beef						■
with chicken						■

FOOD	ALKALINE-FORMING			ACID-FORMING		
	High	Medium	Low	Low	Medium	High
SIDE DISHES						
Baked potato, skin on, plain		■				
French fried onion rings						■
French fried potatoes						■
Green salad (mixed greens), plain		■				
CONDIMENTS AND DRESSINGS						
Catsup (ketchup)					■	
Mayonnaise				■		
Mustard					■	
Salad Dressings						
Caesar						■
French					■	
Italian, with olive oil and apple cider vinegar			■			
Russian				■		
Thousand Island					■	
BEVERAGES						
Coffee, black (regular or decaffeinated)					■	
Milk shake, any flavor						■
Soft drink (carbonated)						■

FOOD	ALKALINE-FORMING			ACID-FORMING		
	High	Medium	Low	Low	Medium	High
Tea						
black, most types				■		
herbal, most types			■			

Water, bottled mineral. *See* Water on page 154.

DESSERTS						
Apple pie						■
Ice cream sundae						■

BREAKFAST DISHES						
Bacon and eggs						■
Biscuits						■
Breakfast sandwich with eggs, cheese, and sausage or ham						■
Hash brown potatoes			■			
Sausage (pork) and eggs						■

GLOSSARY

Acid. Any substance in the body that gives off hydrogen ions when it is dissolved in water. Such substances have a pH value of less than 7.0.

Acid-alkaline balance. A necessary element of health created by a balanced state of acidic and alkaline substances in the body's fluids and tissues.

Acidic. Having a pH value less than 7.0.

Acidifying. Producing an acidic state.

Acidogenic. Acid-producing.

Acidogenic diet. A diet consisting primarily of foods that create an acid load in the body after they are eaten and metabolized.

Acidosis. A state of excessive acidity in the body's tissues and fluids. Acid buildup.

Adenosine triphosphate (ATP). A fuel synthesized by the cells from oxygen and glucose. ATP provides energy for many metabolic processes and is involved in making the genetic material RNA.

Aerobic. A term literally meaning "with oxygen," used in this book to designate an oxygen-rich environment. In the human body, an aerobic state enables the body to defend itself against harmful microorganisms such as bacteria, fungi, and viruses.

Alkali. Any substance that accepts hydrogen ions when it is dissolved in water. Such a substance has a pH value of more than 7.0, and is also referred to as a base.

Alkaline. Having a pH value greater than 7.0.

Alkalizing. Producing an alkaline state.

Alkalosis. A state of excessive alkalinity in the body's tissues and fluids. Although rare, chronic alkalosis can be life threatening.

Amino acid. One of the molecular units used by the body to synthesize proteins. Some amino acids are produced by the body, while others must be provided by the diet.

Anaerobic. A term meaning "without oxygen." In the human body, an anaerobic state is conducive to the growth of harmful microorganisms such as bacteria, fungi, and viruses.

Antioxidant. Any substance that prevents or slows the process of oxidation, which produces cell-damaging free radicals.

ATP. *See* Adenosine triphosphate.

Base. *See* Alkali.

Bicarbonate. The most important buffer in the blood. Bicarbonate is a major alkali (base) that transforms and neutralizes acids by taking on their hydrogen ions.

Catabolic state. A state in which an organism breaks down its own tissues.

Catabolism. The metabolic breakdown of molecules in an organism, often resulting in a release of energy.

Central nervous system. The main information-processing organs of the nervous system, consisting of the brain and spinal cord.

Demineralization. A loss of minerals from the body. In a state of chronic acidity, demineralization occurs when the body uses its stores of calcium, potassium, magnesium, and other alkalizing minerals to buffer acid wastes.

Electrolyte. Any substance which, in liquid form, is capable of conducting an electric current through the body. Acids, bases, and salts are common forms of electrolytes. Electrolytes help regulate fluid levels in the body, maintain proper pH, and play a vital role in the transmission of nerve impulses from the brain to the rest of the body.

Enzyme. A protein substance that acts as a catalyst for chemical reactions within the body. Enzymes are necessary for every activity the body performs each day, including breathing, digestion, immune function, reproduction, and organ function, as well as speech, thought, and movement.

Free radical. An unstable molecule that attacks other molecules, causing them to become free radicals as well. When free radical production becomes excessive, cellular damage occurs, leading to disease.

Genetic predisposition. An increased tendency for either health or disease based on factors passed down from generation to generation through the genes. The term is often used to refer to an increased risk for certain diseases based upon hereditary factors.

HCl. *See* Hydrochloric acid.

Homeostasis. The body's inherent ability and tendency to regulate itself through mechanisms that seek to maintain equilibrium, or balance, within all of the body's systems.

Hormone. A chemical messenger sent from one cell to another to help regulate proper cell and organ function, aid in the body's response to stress, and assist in proper metabolism and energy production.

Hydrion paper. A paper that has been impregnated with a pH-sensitive mixture of indicator dyes. When the strip comes in contact with an acid or base substance, it changes color, with each color indicating a different pH value.

Hydrochloric acid (HCl). An acid secreted by the stomach to break down and help digest food.

Hydrogen ion. A single, unstable proton created when hydrogen molecules are dissolved in water through a process known as dissociation. All acids in the body give off hydrogen ions when they are dissolved in water. pH values are determined by the concentration of hydrogen ions in a substance.

Hydrogen ion concentration. The measurement used

to determine a substance's pH value. The greater the concentration of hydrogen ions in a substance, the more acidic it is, while substances with lesser concentrations are less acidic.

Inflammation. A response of the body's tissues to injury or infection, characterized by redness, heat, swelling, pain, and organ dysfunction.

Ion. An atom or group of atoms that has a positive or negative charge as a result of losing or gaining one or more electrons.

Metabolic acidosis. A state in which the blood pH is low (acidic). This condition can be caused either by an accumulation of excess acids or by abnormal losses of bicarbonate.

Metabolism. The biochemical reactions and interactions within the body that result in the production of energy and nutrients necessary to sustain life. Also, the breakdown of food and its transformation into energy.

Mitochondria. The cells' internal energy factories, which produce a compound called adenosine triphosphate—a fuel that furnishes energy for the body.

Mole. The term used to describe the molecular weight of a substance. pH is determined by measuring the concentration of hydrogen ions, which is calculated as moles per liter.

Molecular weight. *See* Mole.

Molecule. The smallest quantity into which a substance can be reduced without losing any of its characteristics. The smallest molecular structures consist of a single atom, while a combination of two or more atoms creates molecular chemical compounds.

Osteoporosis. A condition in which the bones lose mass and density, becoming more porous and prone to fracture.

Over-acidity. A condition characterized by an excessively high acidic pH.

Over-alkalinity. A condition characterized by an excessively high alkaline pH.

Pathogen. Any form of microorganism, such as bacteria, fungi, or viruses, capable of causing disease.

Peripheral nervous system. The nerves that transmit messages from the spinal cord and brain to other parts of the body.

pH. Literally meaning "potential for hydrogen," a measure of the acidity or alkalinity of a solution. The pH scale runs from 0 to 14, with 7.0 considered neutral. pH values below 7.0 are considered acidic, and pH values above 7.0 are considered alkaline.

Proton. A positively charged particle.

Renal. Of or pertaining to the kidneys.

Tetany. An often painful condition characterized by cramps of the voluntary muscles, especially of the fingers, toes, and face.

BIBLIOGRAPHY

Books

Aihara, Herman. *Acid and Alkaline*. Oroville, CA: George Ohsawa Macrobiotic Foundation, 1986.

Auer, Wolfgang. *The Acid Danger*. North Bergin, NJ: Basic Health Publications, Inc., 2004.

Brown, Susan E. *Better Bones, Better Body*. Second Edition. Los Angeles: Keats Publishing, 2000.

Guerrero, Alex. *In Balance for Life*. Garden City Park, NY: Square One Publishers, 2005.

Guyton, Arthur C., and John E. Hall. *Textbook of Medical Physiology*. Ninth Edition. Philadelphia: W.B. Sanders Company, 1996.

Jaffe, Russell M. *The Alkaline Way: Your Health Restoration*. Sterling, VA: ELISA/ACT Biotechnologies, Inc., 2000.

Morter, Ted. *An Apple a Day*. Rogers, Arkansas: Best Research, Inc, 1997.

Trivieri, Larry, Jr., and John Anderson, Editors. *Alternative Medicine: The Definitive Guide*. Second Edition. Berkeley, CA: Ten Speed Press/Celestial Arts, 2002.

Vasey, Christopher. *The Acid-Alkaline Diet*. Rochester, VT: Healing Arts Press, 1999.

Wang, Sang. *Reverse Aging*. Englewood Cliffs, NJ: Siloam Enterprise, Inc., 1994.

Wiley, Rudolph A. *BioBalance: The Acid/Alkaline Solution to the Food-Mood-Health Puzzle*. Hurricane, UT: Essential Science Publishing, 1989.

Journal Articles and Abstracts

Arnett, T. "Regulation of bone cell function by acid-base balance." *Proceedings of the Nutrition Society* 62(2):511–520, 2003.

Brown, S. and R. Jaffe. "Acid-alkaline balance and its effect on bone health." *International Journal of Integrative Medicine* 2 (6): Nov/Dec 2000.

Buclin, T., M. Cosina, M. Appenzeller, A.F. Jacquet, L.A. Decosterd, J. Biollaz, and P. Burckhardt. "Diet acids and alkalis influence calcium retention in bone." *Osteoporosis International* 12(6): 493–499, 2001.

Bushinsky, D.A. and K.K. Frick. "The effects of acid on bone." *Current Opinion in Nephrology and Hypertension* 9(4):369–379, 2000.

Bushinsky, D.A., S.B. Smith, K.L. Gavrilov, L.F. Gavrilov, J. Li, and R. Levi-Setti. "Chronic acidosis-induced alteration in bone bicarbonate and phosphate." *American Journal of Physiology* 285(3): F532–F539, 2003.

Cseuz, R.M., T. Bender, and J. Vormann. "Alkaline mineral supplementation for patients with rheumatoid arthritis." *Rheumatology* 44 (Supplement 1):i79, 2005.

Disthabanchong, S., S. Domrongkichaiporn, V. Sirikulchayanonta, W. Stitchantrakul, P. Karnsombut, and R. Rajatanavin. "Alteration of noncollagenous bone matrix proteins in distal renal tubular acidosis." *Bone* 35(3):604–613, 2004.

Frassetto, L.A., R.C. Morris, Jr., and A. Sebastian. "Effect of age on blood acid-base composition in adult humans: Role of age-related renal functional decline." *American Journal of Physiology* 271(6 Pt. 2):F1114–F1122, 1996.

Frassetto, L.A., R.C. Morris, Jr., and A. Sebastian. "Potassium bicarbonate reduces urinary nitrogen excretion in postmenopausal women." *Journal of Clinical Endocrinology and Metabolism* 82(1): 254–259, 1997.

Frassetto, L.A., E. Nash, R.C. Morris, Jr., and A. Sebastian. "Comparative effects of potassium chloride and bicarbonate on thiazide-induced reduction in urinary calcium excretion." *Kidney International* 58(2):748–752, 2000.

Frassetto, L.A., K.M. Todd, R.C. Morris, Jr., and A. Sebastian. "Estimation of net endogenous noncarbonic acid production in humans from diet potassium and protein contents." *American Journal of Clinical Nutrition* 68(3):576–583, 1998.

Frassetto, L.A., K.M. Todd, R.C. Morris, Jr., and A. Sebastian. "Worldwide incidence of hip fracture in elderly women: Relation to consumption of animal and vegetable foods." *The Journals of Gerontology, Series A* 55(10):M585–M592, 2000.

Frick, K.K. and D.A. Bushinsky. "Metabolic acidosis stimulates RANKL RNA expression in bone through a cyclo-oxygenase-dependent mechanism." *Journal of Bone and Mineral Research* 18(7):1317–1325, 2003.

Heaney, R.P. "Dietary protein and phosphorus do not affect calcium absorption." *American Journal of Clinical Nutrition* 72(3): 758–761, 2000.

Ince, B.A., E.J. Anderson, and R.M. Neer. "Lowering dietary protein to U.S. recommended dietary allowance levels reduces urinary calcium excretion and bone resorption in young women." *Journal of Clinical Endocrinology and Metabolism* 89(8):3801–3807, 2004.

Lemann, J., Jr., D.A. Bushinsky, and L.L. Hamm. "Bone buffering of acid and base in humans." *American Journal of Physiology* 285(5):F811–F832, 2003.

MacDonald, H.M., S.A. New, M.H. Golden, M.K. Campbell, and D.M. Reid. "Nutritional associations with bone loss during the menopausal transition: Evidence of a beneficial effect of calcium, alcohol, and fruit and vegetable nutrients and of a detrimental effect of fatty acids." *American Journal of Clinical Nutrition* 79(1):155–165, 2004.

Marangella, M., M. Di Stefano, S. Casalis, S. Berutti, P.D. Amelio, and G.C. Isaia. "Effects of potassium citrate supplementation on bone metabolism." *Calcified Tissue International* 74(4):330–335, 2004.

Maurer, M., W. Riesen, J. Muser, H.N. Hulter, and R. Krapf. "Neutralization of Western diet inhibits bone resorption independently of K intake and reduces cortisol secretion in humans." *American Journal of Physiology* 284(1):F32–F40, 2003.

McGartland, C.P., P.J. Robson, L.J. Murray, G.W. Cran, M.J. Savage, D.C. Watkins, M.M. Rooney, and C.A. Boreham. "Fruit and vegetable consumption and bone mineral density: The Northern Ireland Young Hearts Project." *American Journal of Clinical Nutrition* 80(4):1019–1023, 2004.

New, S.A. "Intake of fruit and vegetables: Implications for bone health." *Proceedings of the Nutrition Society* 62(4):889–899, 2003.

New, S.A. "The role of the skeleton in acid-base homeostasis." *Proceedings of the Nutrition Society* 61(2):151–164, 2002.

New, S.A., C. Bolton-Smith, D.A. Grubb, and D.M. Reid. "Nutritional influences on bone mineral density: A cross-sectional study in premenopausal women." *American Journal of Clinical Nutrition* 65(6):1831–1839, 1997.

New, S.A., H.M. MacDonald, M.K. Campbell, J.C. Martin, M.J. Garton, S.P. Robins, and D.M. Reid. "Lower estimates of net endogenous non-carbonic acid production are positively associated with indexes of bone health in premenopausal and perimenopausal women." *American Journal of Clinical Nutrition* 79(1):131–138, 2004.

New, S.A., S.P. Robins, M.K. Campbell, J.C. Martin, M.J. Garton, C. Bolton-Smith, D.A. Grubb, S.J. Lee, and D.M. Reid. "Dietary influences on bone mass and bone metabolism: Further evidence of a positive link between fruit and vegetable consumption and bone health." *American Journal of Clinical Nutrition* 71(1):142–151, 2000.

Prynne, C.J., F. Ginty, A.A. Paul, C. Bolton-Smith, S.J. Stear, S.C. Jones, and A. Prentice. "Dietary acid-base balance and intake of bone-related nutrients in Cambridge teenagers." *European Journal of Clinical Nutrition* 58(11):1462–1471, 2004.

Queen, Sam. "Free radical therapy: Part IV—acidemia and free calcium excess." *Health Realities* 13(4): 1994.

Reddy, S.T., C.Y. Wang, K. Sakhaee, L. Brinkley, and C.Y.C. Pak. "Effect of low-carbohydrate high-protein diets on acid-base balance, stone-forming propensity, and calcium metabolism." *American Journal of Kidney Diseases* 40(2):265–274, 2002.

Remer, T. "Influence of diet on acid-base balance." *Seminars in Dialysis* 13(4):221–226, 2000.

Remer, T., T. Dimitriou, and F. Manz. "Dietary potential renal acid load and renal net acid excretion in healthy, free-living children and adolescents." *American Journal of Clinical Nutrition* 77(5):1255–1260, 2003.

Remer, T. and F. Manz. "Estimation of the renal net acid excretion by adults consuming diets containing variable amounts of proteins." *American Journal of Clinical Nutrition* 59(6): 1356–1361, 1994.

Remer, T. and F. Manz. "Paleolithic diet, sweet potato eaters, and potential renal acid load." Letter to the Editor, *American Journal of Clinical Nutrition* 78(4): 802–803, 2003.

Remer, T. and F. Manz. "Potential renal acid load of foods and its influence on urine pH." *Journal of the American Dietetic Association* 95(7):791–797, 1995.

Sebastian, A., S.T. Harris, J.H. Ottaway, K.M. Todd, and R.C. Morris, Jr. "Improved mineral balance and skeletal metabolism in postmenopausal women treated with potassium bicarbonate." *New England Journal of Medicine* 330(25):1776–1781, 1994.

Sebastian, A., L.A. Frassetto, D.E. Sellmeyer, R.L. Merriam, and R.C. Morris, Jr. "Estimation of the net acid load of the diet of ancestral preagricultural *Homo sapiens* and their hominid ancestors." *American Journal of Clinical Nutrition* 76(6):1308–1316, 2002.

Sellmeyer, D.E., K.L. Stone, A. Sebastian, and S.R. Cummings.

"A high ratio of dietary animal to vegetable protein increases the rate of bone loss and the risk of fracture in postmenopausal women." *American Journal of Clinical Nutrition* 73(1):118–122, 2001.

Tucker, K.L., M.T. Hannan, H. Chen, L.A. Cupples, P.W. Wilson, and D.P. Kiel. "Potassium, magnesium, and fruit and vegetable intakes are associated with greater bone mineral density in elderly men and women." *American Journal of Clinical Nutrition* 69(4):727–736, 1999.

Vaitkevicius, H., R. Witt, M. Maasdam, K. Walters, M. Gould, S. Mackenzie, S. Farrow, and W. Lockette. "Ethnic differences in titratable acid excretion and bone mineralization." *Medicine and Science in Sports and Exercise* 34(2):295–302, 2002.

Vormann, J. and D. Hannelore. "Acid-base metabolism. Nutrition, health, disease." Editorial, *European Journal of Nutrition* 40(5):187–189, 2001.

Vormann, J., M. Worlitschek, T. Goedecke, and B. Silver. "Supplementation with alkaline minerals reduces symptoms in patients with chronic low back pain." *Journal of Trace Elements in Medicine & Biology* 15(2-3):179–183, 2001.

Whiting, S.J., J. Bell, and S. Brown. "First morning urine measured with pH strip reflects acid excretion." Research abstract presented at the American Society of Bone and Mineral Research (ASBMR), San Antonio, Texas, 2002.

Wiederkehr, M. and R. Krapf. "Metabolic and endocrine effects of metabolic acidosis in humans." *Swiss Medical Weekly* 131 (9–10):127–132, 2001.

Zwart, S.R., A.R. Hargens, and S.M. Smith. "The ratio of animal protein intake to potassium intake is a predictor of bone resorption in space flight analogues and in ambulatory subjects." *American Journal of Clinical Nutrition* 80(4):1058–1065, 2004.

ALKALIZING SUPPLEMENTS

Alkalizing products—which come in many forms, including powders, capsules, drops, and teas—can enhance the shift from over-acidity to an appropriate acid-alkaline balance. What follows is a list of some of the companies that provide effective pH-balancing products. Be aware that these products should *not* be used as a substitute for an alkaline diet. But if used in conjunction with a sound eating plan, as described in Chapter 4, they can help speed your way to health. After one or two weeks of daily use, be sure to test your pH as detailed in Chapter 3. This will help you evaluate the progress you have made. Based upon your individual body chemistry, you may find that one product works better for you than another. Don't be afraid to change products if you find that the one you've been taking is not helping you reach your goal of a healthy pH balance.

Barlean's Organic Oils, L.L.C.
4936 Lake Terrell Road
Ferndale, Washington 98248
Phone: 360-384-0485
Website: www.barleans.com

Both Barlean's Greens powder and Barlean's Greens capsules contain alkalizing green foods, which provide minerals, vitamins, fiber, enzymes, carotenoids, and antioxidants.

Chi's Enterprise
P.O. Box 753
Atwood, CA 92811
Phone: 714-777-1542
Website: www.chi-health.com

Asparagus Extract is a powdered concentrate of the whole asparagus plant, which has been grown organically. It is available in capsules and tea bags.

Jarrow Formulas
1824 S. Robertson Boulevard
Los Angeles, CA 90035
Phone: 800-726-0886
Website: www.jarrow.com

Jarrow Formulas offers three alkalizing products. Yaeyama Chlorella, which contains the fresh water algae chlorella, comes in powder, capsule, and tablet form. Yaeyama Chlorella + Barley is a barley-chlorella combination in tablet form. Green Defense is a phytonutrient-rich green vegetable powder.

Mt. Capra Whole Food Nutritionals
279 SW 9th Street
Chehalis, WA 98532
Phone: 360-748-4224
Website: www.mtcapra.com

Capra Mineral Whey is a high-potassium dehydrated goat milk whey that contains more than twenty naturally occurring minerals.

Nature's Brands
6 September Circle
E. Stroudsburg, PA 18301
Phone: 888-417-1375
Website: www.NaturallyDirect.net

Nature's Brands offers two products. Acid-2-Alkaline, an all-natural vegetarian alkalizing formula, is available in capsule, powder, and drop form. Super Herbal Greens, available in capsules and powder, is an alkalizing formula made from thirty different greens.

NOW
395 S. Glen Ellyn Road
Bloomingdale, IL 60108
Website: www.nowfoods.com

Available in both powder and tablet form, Green Phyto-Foods contains phytonutrient-rich products derived from green plants, algae, and cereal grasses.

PERQUE, LLC
14 Pidgeon Hill Drive, Suite 180
Sterling, VA 20165
Phone: 800-525-7372
Website: www.perque.com

Perque offers five alkalizing products. Mg Plus Guard capsules contain a mixture of three ionized alkaline forms of magnesium. Potent C Guard is a highly alkalizing buffered powder containing Vitamin C and alkaline forms of potassium, calcium, magnesium, and zinc. Endura/PAK Guard capsules provide an L-glutamine/alphaketoglutarate formula. Choline Citrate is a liquid formula of pure choline that enhances uptake of magnesium. Bone Guard Forté tablets contain an alkalizing mineral formula.

Peter Gillham's Natural Vitality
4867 Fountain Avenue
Los Angeles, CA 90029
Phone: 800-446-7462
Website: www.ThetaVites.com

Natural Calm and Natural Calm Plus Calcium are both water-soluble powders. Natural Calm provides a highly absorbable form of magnesium, while Natural Calm Plus Calcium provides magnesium plus calcium, vitamin C, vitamin D, and boron.

pH Sciences, Inc.
P.O. Box 65260
Seattle, WA 98155
Phone: 877-363-2243
Website: www.phsciences.com

pH Balance contains an alkalizing blend of potassium, magnesium, and calcium in tablet form.

Phion Nutrition
7741 E. Gray Road, Suite 9
Scottsdale, AZ 85260
Phone: 888-744-8589
Website: www.ph-ion.com

This company offers three products. Alkalive Blue supplement powder contains calcium, magnesium, potassium, manganese, and iron, which help replenish mineral reserves. Alkalive Green supplement powder is composed of dehydrated juices from alkalizing green grasses. Alkalive pH Booster drops include seventy-two ionic minerals that alkalize drinking water to a pH of 9.5.

Premier Research Labs
2000 N. Mays, Suite 120
Round Rock, TX 78664
Phone: 800-325-7734
Website: www.prlabs.com

Quantum Coral Legend contains pure Sango marine coral powder, high in ionized magnesium and calcium. Quantum Aloe Powder provides organic aloe vera leaf powder plus pomegranate powder.

Source Naturals
19 Janis Way
Scotts Valley, CA 95066
Phone: 800-815-2333
Website: www.sourcenaturals.com

Alka-Balance tablets contain an alkalizing blend of nutrients, including calcium, magnesium, sodium, and potassium.

Swanson Health Products
P.O. Box 2803
Fargo, ND 58108-2803
Phone: 800-824-4491
Website: www.swansonvitamins.com

Swanson offers several alkalizing products. The Swanson pH Balance Alkalizing Formula is a drink mix that contains an herbal blend, formulated to help the body maintain a healthy acid-base balance. Alka Fizz, available in tablet form, is designed to tame excess stomach acidity. Apricot Alkalizing Tea helps support and correct body chemistry.

TriMedica International, Inc.
1895 South Los Feliz Drive
Tempe, AZ 85281
Phone: 800-800-8849
Website: www.trimedica.com

Tri-Medica's AlkaMAX supplement line includes both capsules and an effervescent powder designed to restore pH balance.

Växa International
4010 W. State Street
Tampa, FL 33609
Phone: 877-622-8292
Website: www.vaxa.com

Växa's Buffer-pH+ capsules contain a homeopathic formula with natural alkalizing agents.

ORDERING INFORMATION

The pH Hydrion Test Paper

The ph Hydrion Test Paper was designed to measure urine and saliva pH. Each roll is 15 feet long and provides for 100 to 120 pH tests. This special paper measures pH in twelve .2-unit gradients from 5.5 to 8.0, and allows for easy detection of the desired 6.5 to 7.5 pH range.

Price: $13.95 for one roll $24.95 for two rolls (includes shipping)

The Better Bones, Better Body pH Test Kit

This kit contains pH Hydrion Test Paper (described above), The Importance of the Alkaline Diet handout, How to Optimize Your Biochemistry Through Diet, Meals for Better Bones and Better Body pH Balance, selected articles on pH and bone health, and Better Bones, Better Body audio tape interview with Dr. Susan Brown.

Price: $29.95 (includes shipping)

Using the form below, order by mail:
Nutrition Education and Consulting Service
605 Franklin Park Drive, East Syracuse, NY 13057
Order by fax: 315-432-9231. • Order by phone (toll free):
888-206-7119. • Order online: www.alkalineforlife.com.

ORDER FORM

Name _____

Address_____ Apt._____

City_____ State_____ Zip_____

Credit Card # _____ Exp. Date_____

Signature_____

ITEM	QUANTITY	PRICE	TOTAL
		Subtotal	
Sales Tax (New York State residents only) 8% *(Shipping charges are included in the price.)*			
Total enclosed (Enclose check, credit card information, or money order in US funds only.)			

ABOUT THE AUTHORS

Susan E. Brown, PhD, CCN, medical anthropologist and certified nutritionist, has consulted widely on socioeconomic, cultural, educational, and health issues. She has taught in North and South American universities, and has written numerous academic and popular articles. She is also the author of *Better Bones, Better Body: A Comprehensive Self-Help Program for Preventing, Halting & Overcoming Osteoporosis*, and co-author of *The Mend Clinic Guide to Natural Medicine for Menopause and Beyond*.

Currently, Dr. Brown directs the Osteoporosis Education Project and the Nutrition Education and Consulting Service in Syracuse, New York. With the osteoporosis project, she conducts primary research, lectures widely on osteoporosis reversal, and teaches the use of a holistic, natural program for the regeneration of bone health. The Nutrition Education and Consulting Service (NECS) provides consulting, education, research, and lecture services for health professionals and the public, as well as long-distance nutrition consultations by telephone.

In addition to running a busy private practice, Dr. Brown serves as consultant to various medical and industry groups, including Technical Sourcing International, Lane Labs, Natural Option Corporation, pH Sciences, Inc., Seraphim, Inc., ELISA/ACT Biotechnologies, and PR-Osteo.

Dr. Brown received her PhD from the University of Michigan in 1972, and is the recipient of two Fulbright-Hays Scholar Awards, and an Organization of American States Research Fellowship. She is also a member of Sigma Xi, the honorary Scientific Research Organization of North America. Since the fall of 2002, Dr. Brown has served as a research associate at the Department of Anthropology, Syracuse University. You can visit her websites at: www.susanbrownphd.com, www.betterbones.com, and www.alkalineforlife.com.

Larry Trivieri, Jr. has been exploring natural and holistic healing methods for more than thirty years, and is a nationally recognized writer and journalist in the field of holistic and alternative medicine. In addition to writing numerous articles in many leading popular health magazines, Trivieri is the author of *Health on the Edge: Visionary Views of Healing in the New Millennium* and *The American Holistic Medical Association Guide to Holistic Health;* and co-author of *Juice Alive; Chronic Fatigue, Fibromyalgia, and Lyme Disease;* and *The Complete Self-Care Guide to Holistic Medicine.* He is also the editor and co-author of the landmark reference text *Alternative Medicine: The Definitive Guide.*

In 2002, Trivieri founded the comprehensive online resource www.1healthyworld.com and is the publisher of its free online newsletter *The Health Plus Letter,* which is read by subscribers in more than thirty countries. A popular guest on radio and TV shows, Trivieri also lectures nationwide on the subject of health, with an emphasis on empowering self-care approaches that can be used to improve well-being. He resides in his hometown of Utica, New York.

INDEX

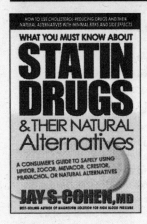

WHAT YOU MUST KNOW ABOUT STATIN DRUGS & THEIR NATURAL ALTERNATIVES

A Consumer's Guide to Safely Using Lipitor, Zocor, Mevacor, Crestor, Pravachol, or Natural Alternatives

Jay S. Cohen, MD

It is estimated that over 100 million Americans suffer from elevated cholesterol and C-reactive proteins—markers that are linked to heart attack, stroke, and other cardiovascular disorders. To combat these problems, modern science has created a group of drugs known either as statins or as specific commercial drugs such as Lipitor, Zocor, and Pravachol. While over 20 million people take these medications, the fact is that up to 42 percent experience side effects, and a whopping 60 to 75 percent eventually stop treatment. Here, for the first time, is a guide that explains the problems caused by statins, and offers easy-to-follow strategies that will allow you to benefit from these drugs while avoiding their side effects. In addition, the author discusses natural alternatives that have also proven effective.

What You Must Know About Statin Drugs & Their Natural Alternatives begins by explaining elevated cholesterol and C-reactive proteins. It then examines how statins work to alleviate these problems, and discusses possible side effects. Highlighted is information on safe usage, as well as a discussion of effective alternative treatments. If you have elevated cholesterol or C-reactive protein levels, or if you are currently using a statin, *What You Must Know About Statin Drugs & Their Natural Alternatives* can make a profound difference in the quality of your life.

$15.95 • 224 pages • 6 x 9-inch paperback • ISBN 0-7570-0257-9

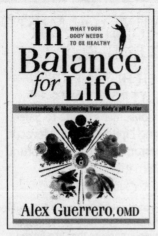

IN BALANCE FOR LIFE

Understanding & Maximizing Your Body's pH Factor

Alex Guerrero

The principle of balance is not new. It forms the very foundation of both Eastern and Western philosophies, from Aristotle to Confucius. As it relates to health, it has been around just as long, from the development of traditional Chinese medicine to the treatments used by Hippocrates and Galen. What is new, however, is a scientifically based application that can improve numerous disorders and maximize your health.

Imagine that the human body has an internal mechanism that keeps two basic types of chemicals—acid and alkali—in balance. When your body becomes either too acidic or too alkaline, you become susceptible to a host of disorders. When balance is restored, however, so is your health. In this brilliant book, renowned health expert Alex Guerrero explains how you can become well—now and for an extended lifetime—by restoring your pH balance. The author first describes how you can assess your health. He then provides a plan, including a fourteen-day diet and a simple program of supplements, that will bring your body back into balance. You'll even find a selection of recipes that will tempt your taste buds as you reclaim your health and well-being.

In Balance for Life offers a revolutionary look at why we become ill. It also presents the simple steps you can follow—each and every day—to enjoy boundless vitality and optimal well-being.

$15.95 • 192 Pages • 6 x 9-inch quality paperback • ISBN 0-7570-0264-1

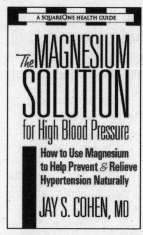

A SQUAREONE HEALTH GUIDE

The MAGNESIUM SOLUTION for High Blood Pressure

How to Use Magnesium to Help Prevent & Relieve Hypertension Naturally

JAY S. COHEN, MD

THE MAGNESIUM SOLUTION FOR HIGH BLOOD PRESSURE

How to Use Magnesium to Prevent & Relieve Hypertension Naturally

Jay S. Cohen, MD

More than 50 million Americans have high blood pressure—a devastating disease that can lead to heart attacks and strokes. Doctors routinely prescribe drugs for this condition, but these medications frequently cause side effects. As a nationally recognized expert on medications and side effects, Dr. Jay S. Cohen wants to make you aware of a safe, natural solution to high blood pressure—the mineral magnesium.

Magnesium is essential for the normal functioning of nerves, muscles, blood vessels, bones, and the heart, yet more than 75% of the population is deficient in it. Dr. Cohen has written *The Magnesium Solution for High Blood Pressure* to provide you and your doctor with all of the information needed to understand why magnesium is essential for helping to prevent and treat high blood pressure. Dr. Cohen explains why magnesium is necessary for normal vascular functioning, how to use magnesium along with hypertension drugs, and the best types of magnesium to use. Most importantly, Dr. Cohen has made the evidence-based research on magnesium's safety and effectiveness highly readable and usable by anyone.

$5.95 • 96 pages • 4 x 7-inch mass paperback • ISBN 0-7570-0255-2

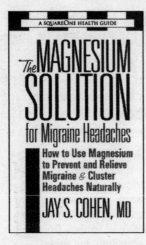

THE MAGNESIUM SOLUTION FOR MIGRAINE HEADACHES

How to Use Magnesium to Prevent and Relieve Migraine & Cluster Headaches Naturally

Jay S. Cohen, MD

More than 30 million people across North America suffer from migraine headaches. Over the years, a number of drugs have been developed to treat migraines, but these treatments don't work for everyone, and come with a high risk of side effects. Fortunately, Dr. Jay S. Cohen has discovered an alternative—magnesium.

This easy-to-understand guide explains what a migraine is, and shows how this supplement can play a key role in preventing and treating migraine headaches. It also describes what type of magnesium works best, and how much magnesium should be taken to prevent or stop migraines. For those who are looking for a safe and effective approach to the prevention and treatment of migraine and cluster headaches, Dr. Cohen prescribes a proven natural remedy in *The Magnesium Solution for Migraine Headaches*.

$5.95 • 96 pages • 4 x 7-inch mass paperback • ISBN 0-7570-0256-0